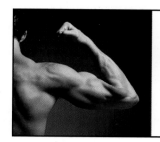

BODYSMART

THE PAIN-FREE WAY TO STAY IN SHAPE

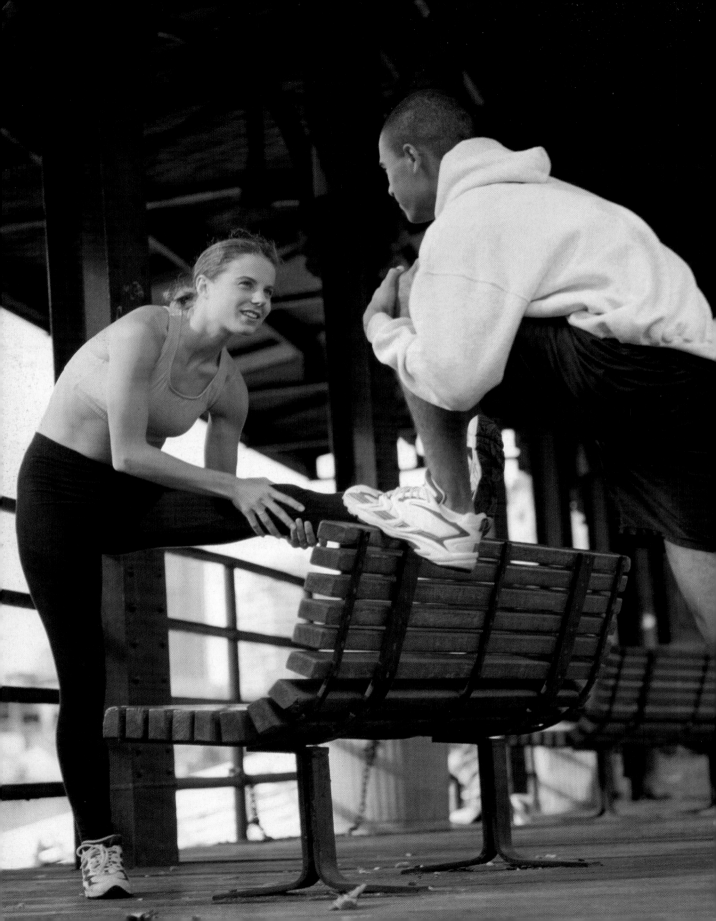

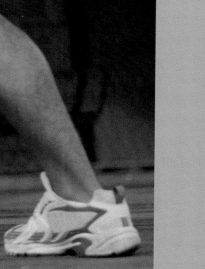

BODYSMART

THE PAIN-FREE WAY TO STAY IN SHAPE

NICK WOOLLEY

Carroll & Brown Publishers Limited

This book is dedicated to the loving memory of my late father.

First published in 2004 in the United Kingdom by

Carroll & Brown Publishers Limited
20 Lonsdale Road
London NW6 6RD

Project Editors: Kirsten Chapman, Anna Amari-Parker
Designer: Jim Cheatle
Production: Karol Davies
Computer Management: Paul Stradling

Text and illustrations © Nick Woolley 2004
Additional illustrations and compilation © Carroll & Brown Limited 2004

A CIP catalogue record for this book is available from the British Library.

ISBN 1-903258-80-4

10 9 8 7 6 5 4 3 2 1

Reproduced in Singapore by Colourscan
Printed in Italy by STIGE Turin

Contents

Introduction

Only 30 years ago, the gym was a place for men—and the occasional woman—to get bigger and stronger, healthy eating was a big steak, and people would take whatever the doctor prescribed without question. In recent years, we have become far more aware of the role that health and fitness play in our lives.

Encouraged by the media and the health and fitness industry, we now devote more time to ourselves. Increased public awareness and an upsurge in the material available on such topics means most of us now have a better idea of how to look after ourselves mentally and physically. Gyms and health clubs are now filled with people of all ages from all walks of life. In much the same way, aspects of the field of medicine that were once dismissed as quackery are now widely accepted components of mainstream medical practice. As more and more people become disillusioned with blindly taking pills, we are gradually turning back toward natural remedies and treatments.

Top sportspeople are generally bigger, stronger, and faster. They now have access to vastly improved training facilities and knowledge, because in the competitive world of sports, even the smallest of margins can spell the difference between success and failure.

Posture and pain-relief

However, for many people the role of posture in maintaining health and physical capability has been largely overlooked. If your body's postural stability is violated, your muscles have to work harder to counteract the negative responses that follow. If your body is out of balance, your physical performance can be affected and you will often start to feel pain. In fact, many people have seemingly inexplicable pains that are the result of tight muscles and distortions.

If you are trying to run faster or throw farther, you will never reach your peak potential, no matter how hard you train your muscles and perfect your technique. Likewise, if you are trying to relieve pain and discomfort without first addressing the underlying postural and biomechanical issues, you may find that you can't get rid of the problem or that it keeps on coming back.

A different approach

During many years of study, I often found it difficult to source the information I was looking for. There was never one teacher who had all the answers to my questions. This spurred me on to approach my studies of the human body and the way it adapts to the things we do from different angles. Instead of trying to find one all-encompassing treatment or therapy, I decided to look at all the variables that occurred when the body was injured or not functioning properly.

This is a little like looking at a soccer team in action: although there are several positions that you can play and each position requires its own unique set of skills, the team can only function as a complete unit if they all come together.

Similarly, there are different "positions" that the human body has in response to mechanical dysfunction. Muscles can become tight or weak, and the body's soft tissues (muscles, tendons, ligaments, and fascia) can affect posture and function or be affected by posture and function. I started to investigate which techniques and

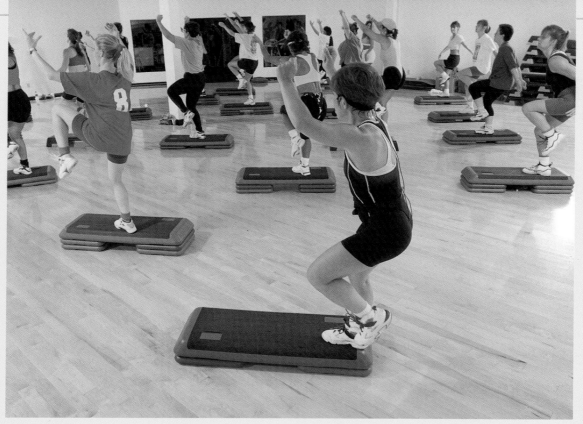

Good posture and balance are the foundations of overall health and well-being.

therapies worked best for each "position" and began to match them up or combine them. Some techniques specialized on weakened muscles, some on tightened muscles, some on stretching, and some on strengthening. When I had pieced them all together, I obtained the winning formula for *BodySmart*.

What the book offers

BodySmart presents a clear, concise path to a healthy, pain-free body. It is intended to bridge the gap between what you know and don't know about your body. The information and techniques in this book stem from various sources, including rehabilitation therapies, as well as my own personal and professional research and observations as a sports therapist and athlete. They will be beneficial not only to people suffering from pain and discomfort, but also to sportspeople, fitness trainers, coaches, therapists, students of physical education, and

those of you simply wishing to improve your flexibility and general health.

This book is aimed at anyone who has ever wanted to learn more about improving the performance and well-being of his or her body. Structural body mapping will show you how to "read" your body, so you can recognize and rectify those imbalances that may be preventing you from reaching your true physical potential. *BodySmart* will guide you to an understanding of how your body works, how to look after it, how to maximize its performance, and how to spot when it is not functioning properly. Whether to relieve pain and discomfort, improve flexibility and posture, for sporting purposes or just to enjoy the incredible sense of vitality that a well-functioning body gives you, *BodySmart* was written for you.

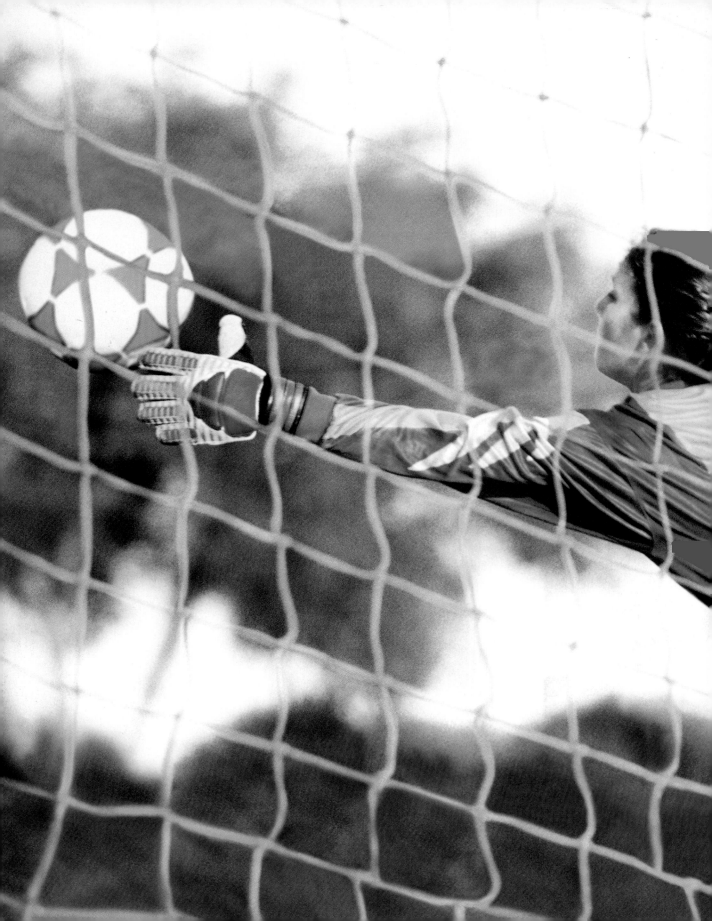

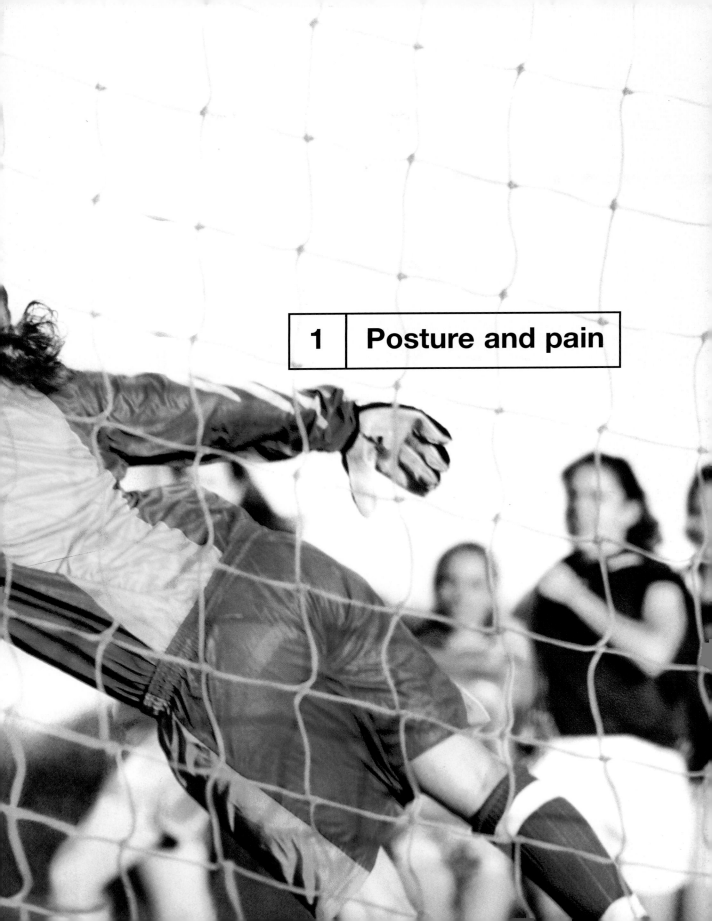

1 | Posture and pain

The musculoskeletal system

Before looking at what your body does and why it does it, take a moment to consider what goes into making you "you." This section provides an overview of your body's nuts and bolts—your anatomy. Familiarize yourself with how you are built and gain the knowledge to take control of your body.

Your physical structure is responsible for stability and movement. This section examines bones, joints, ligaments, muscles, and tendons and how they connect and function.

Bones

You are born with over 350 bones in your body, though many join together as you mature. The largest number of bones are found in your spine (33), the hands and feet (26 each including the wrists and ankles), and the head (another 26 including the skull and face).

Your skeleton is divided into two groups. The bones in the axial skeleton—consisting of your skull, vertebral column, breastbone (sternum), and ribs—form your central core. Their fairly rigid structure supports your body and helps contain and protect your delicate internal organs, brain, and spinal cord. The bones in the appendicular skeleton—the shoulder blades (scapulae), collarbones (clavicles), pelvis, arms, wrists, hands, legs, ankles, and feet—are collectively not as rigid as those of the axial skeleton, and are key to movement and locomotion.

As the hardest part of the body, bones may look like dry, rigid, lumps of wood but they are actually living, growing tissue. With the exception of your skull, each bone is encased in its

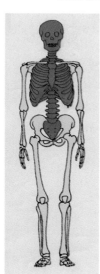

The axial skeleton (shaded brown) is at your core. The appendicular skeleton (shaded yellow) enables movement.

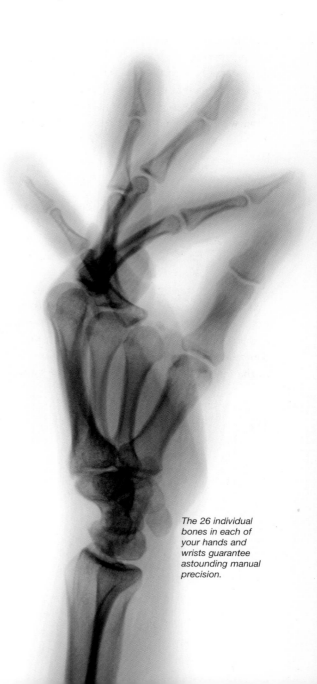

The 26 individual bones in each of your hands and wrists guarantee astounding manual precision.

own protective sheath (the periosteum). This layer supplies the bone with blood and special bone-developing cells, which help the bone grow and heal if it gets damaged. If you are unlucky enough to break or fracture a bone, your body will quickly get to work on mending it by growing new bone tissue around the injured area.

Building bone density

Bones adapt to increased loads by becoming stronger. For this reason, weightlifters generally have far greater bone tissue density than the average person. Regular exercise—especially using some type of resistance (e.g. weight training or stair-climbing)—helps keep bones strong and healthy. T'ai chi and yoga are also good ways of strengthening bones, as the slow movements they involve place firm, yet safe, levels of stress on the bones.

Joints

The points at which two bones meet are known as joints, and these are what make movement possible. The body contains three main types of joints, classified by how much movement they allow. Fibrous joints (e.g. between the bones of the skull) are closely connected bones, which may even be fused. Cartilaginous joints provide very limited movement, such as between the right and left sides of the pelvis. Finally, the most common type are the synovial joints. Some, such as the knee and elbow—known as hinge joints—

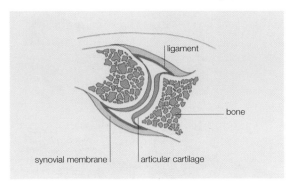

Cross-section of a synovial joint

can move in only two directions, but ball-and-socket joints, such as in the shoulder or hip, can be rotated through nearly 360 degrees. Synovial joints are freely moveable and surrounded by synovial fluid, which lubricates the surfaces of the bones and acts as a shock absorber.

Ligaments

Bands of tough, fibrous tissue, known as ligaments fasten two bones together to form a strong and stable joint. These attachments allow the joint to act like a pivot around which movement can occur. To understand the mechanics of this, consider how the doors in your home are fitted into their doorframes. Without their hinges, they would come crashing down every time they were opened. Hinges effectively stop doors from falling out of their frames while making movement possible. Your ligaments act like hinges to keep your bones secure and stable once movement begins within the joints. Ligaments also control the range of

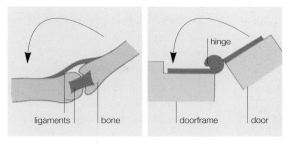

The hinge principle underpinning ligament-bone action in joints

movement that takes place so the bones do not move too far apart and damage the joints. Those individuals who are considered to be double-jointed haven't actually got double joints as such, but simply have looser ligaments that allow for a greater range of movement within the joint.

Muscles

Of all the structures in the human body, muscles are the most abundant. Some 40 percent of your body weight comes from your muscles. As well as giving you movement and strength, muscles pad you out to give you your recognizable size and shape. In addition to what we normally think of as "muscles," there are two specialized types of tissue: cardiac muscle, which functions without conscious control and is found only in your heart; and smooth muscle, which lines areas such as the blood vessels and digestive tracts and which also tends to function involuntarily.

You have about 650 muscles in total, each with the ability to contract and relax. It is this contraction-relaxation dynamic that enables you to move. Your standard (skeletal) muscles are made up of bundles of cells known as fibers. When a muscle tenses, the individual fibers contract and shorten, bringing the ends of the muscle closer together. This moves the bone to which that muscle is attached (see 1 below). In order to return the bone back to its starting position, the contracted muscle relaxes while its opposing muscle contracts (see 2 below). This simple sequence of contraction and relaxation gives you the ability to walk, run, sit, and stand.

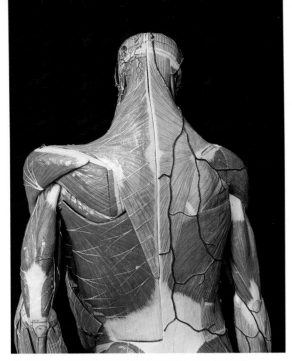

An anatomy model showing back muscles, blood vessels (red/blue), tendons/ligaments (white), and bones (cream).

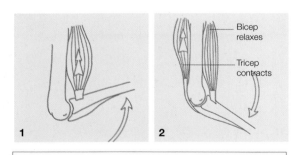

Muscle speak: There are several terms that health/fitness professionals use when discussing muscles. The term "agonist" refers to the muscle that contracts. The "antagonist" is the opposing, relaxing muscle. In example 1, the bicep is the agonist. In example 2, the tricep is the agonist, and the bicep the antagonist.

Skeletal muscles can't contract or relax of their own accord but need to be "told" to do so. It is a little like a light being turned on. When you flip the switch, an electrical current is passed through the wires into the light. This electrical energy heats up the filament inside the bulb, causing it to glow. Your muscles, too, need an electrical impulse to move. This signal comes from the brain and is carried along your nerves—the body's version of electric wires—into the muscle, causing the fibers to contract. The stronger the impulse, the greater the number of fibers that contract and the greater the strength of that contraction. The opposite effect is also true: the weaker the signal, the fewer fibers contract and the weaker the movement.

Increasing muscular strength

Just like bone, if muscles are forced to work harder and against more resistance than they are accustomed to, the fibers become stronger and larger. This is called hypertrophy, from the Greek words hyper, meaning "over" or "beyond" and trophia, meaning "nourishment." Such muscular enlargement is evident in body builders and strength athletes as they train by lifting increasingly heavier weights.

Conversely, if muscles are not worked at all, the muscle fibers start to shrink and atrophy, from the Greek a, meaning "not" and trophia, "nourishment." This reduction in muscle size can best be seen when a cast is first removed after a broken bone has mended. During convalescence, all muscle movement is prohibited and a shrinkage in size by as much as 25 percent can occur in the first 48 hours.

Keeping your body reasonably fit and giving your muscles some kind of resistance to work against is very beneficial. It helps keep your muscles strong and healthy, increases the strength of your ligaments and tendons, improves the strength and health of your joints, and encourages general circulation.

Tendons

Connecting muscles to bones are strong cord-like structures called tendons. These strands of connective tissue are extensions of the muscle fibers found at the ends of each muscle. Tendons, unlike muscles, cannot contract, although they do have a small degree of elasticity to them. At one end, the tendon merges into the muscle; at the other, it connects to the bone via the periosteum.

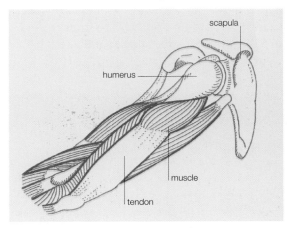

Cross-section of the layout of muscles and tendons around the shoulder blade (scapula) and the upper arm (humerus).

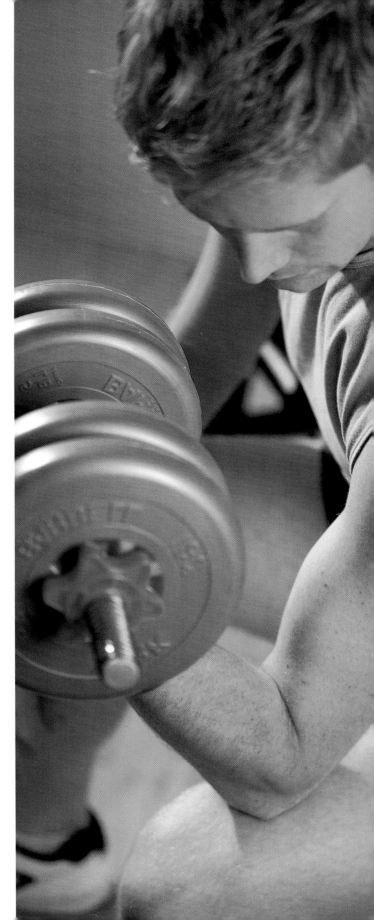

The skeletal muscles

These diagrams provide an overview of the musculo-skeletal system, showing some of the key muscles involved in maintaining your posture.

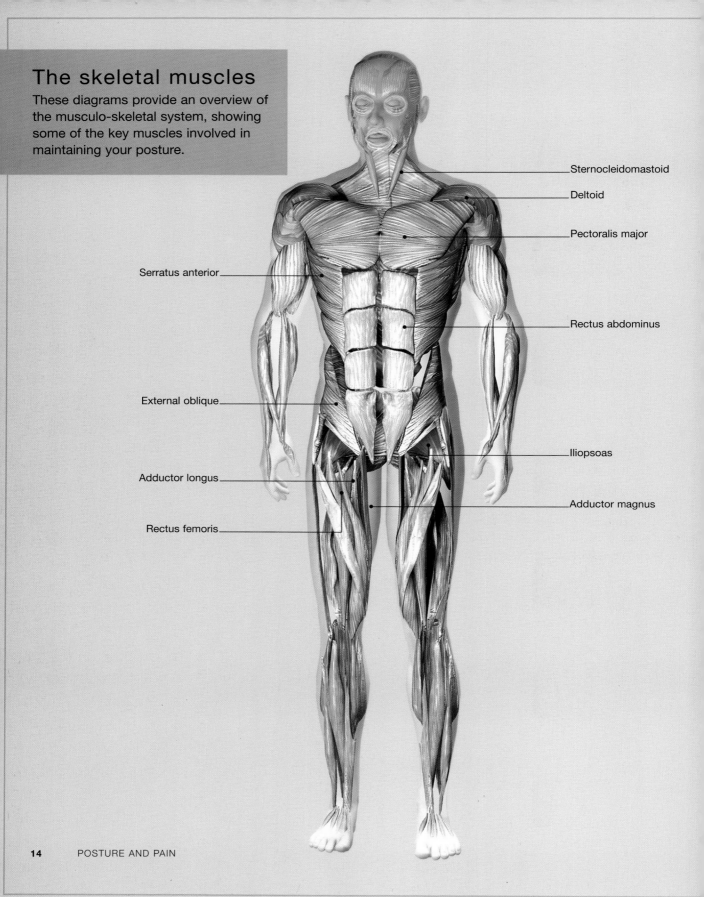

Sternocleidomastoid

Deltoid

Pectoralis major

Serratus anterior

Rectus abdominus

External oblique

Iliopsoas

Adductor longus

Adductor magnus

Rectus femoris

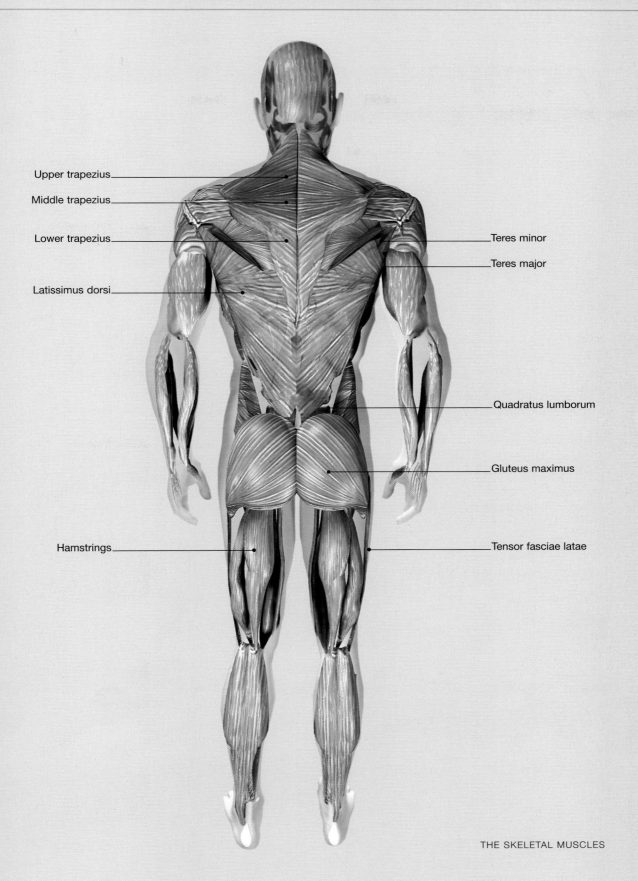

Upper trapezius

Middle trapezius

Lower trapezius

Latissimus dorsi

Hamstrings

Teres minor

Teres major

Quadratus lumborum

Gluteus maximus

Tensor fasciae latae

The mechanics of muscle action

There are a few concepts that can help you understand how your muscles work and what can go wrong: firstly, your muscles are always partially contracted, even when you are asleep; secondly, each muscle has a certain length and a certain degree of flexibility; thirdly, your muscles work in pairs.

Your muscles always contain a minimum amount of healthy tension, even when you are completely relaxed. This tension is known as your natural muscle tone. Each of your muscles also has a certain length and degree of flexibility that it should be able to maintain naturally. If a muscle becomes chronically tight and starts to shorten, it loses this ability and its muscle tone increases. It is this increased muscle tone that can start to pull your body out of alignment.

Muscle pairs

For every muscle that does one thing, you have another muscle that does the opposite. The muscles at the front of your thigh that allow you to straighten your leg, for example, are complemented by muscles at the back of your thigh that allow you to bend it back again. Where you have muscles that allow you to push, you also have opposing muscles that allow you to pull. Any movement you make has a countermovement: you can push and pull; you can raise and lower; you can twist to the left and to the right; and so on.

The key to good posture and correct biomechanics lies in the interaction between opposing muscles. When a muscle shortens in length, it moves the position of the bone to which it is connected. Therefore, if the muscles that lift your shoulder up, for example, are tighter and have a greater tension than those muscles responsible for pulling your shoulder

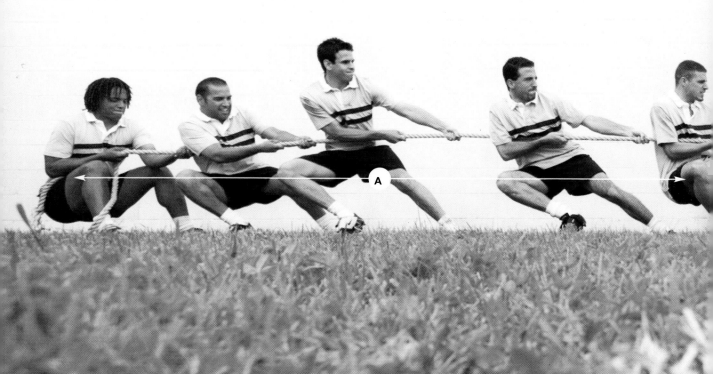

A

down, your shoulder will be held in a raised and mechanically incorrect position.

Natural tension

The natural tension between opposing muscles creates a kind of tug-of-war. As long as both muscles are an equal match, they can mutually resist each other's pull and maintain a balance. But when one muscle becomes stronger than the other and its muscle tone increases, it can overpower its equivalent. This unequal force shortens the stronger muscle and increases the pull on the bone to which it is attached. If the imbalance is considerable, the bone may be shifted away from its natural position to such an extent that a noticeable distortion occurs.

Imagine a tug-of-war between two teams, team A and team B (see picture below). Think of them as opposing muscles with the knot in the middle of the rope (1) representing the stability of a bone or joint. If A and B generate the same amount of strength—say 1000 lbs (454 kg) of force—they will counter each other's influence. This balance represents the ideal relationship between two muscles, where a stable postural position is maintained because of equal muscle tone.

But if A pulls harder, generating 1500 lbs (682 kg) of force, while B produces only 1000 lbs (454 kg) of force, an imbalance will occur. Team A will start to move backward, causing the center of the rope to shift toward the stronger side. In terms of muscle dynamics, A would be the cause of movement, because as the muscle tightens, its muscle tone increases and its pulling capacity draws the bone out of its natural position. Good posture is thus compromised.

There is another way in which the same distortion can take place. If team A's effort does not increase, but remains constant at 1000 lbs (454 kg) and B reduces its pulling strength to 500 lbs (227 kg), team A will still end up exerting greater strength in relation to B. The end result is the same: team A moves backward and the knot once again moves to the left. In muscle terms, as the tone of the opposing muscle, B, decreases, the relative muscle tone of A increases, causing it to once again become tight and restricted. It is a major misconception that tight muscles are always the cause of distortion in themselves.

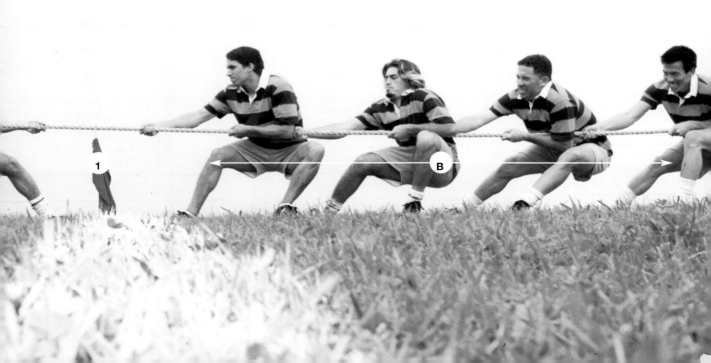

Posture

Your body's mechanical integrity is the very cornerstone of its physical health and wellbeing. Good posture is conducive to strength, agility, and unrestricted movement, whereas bad posture results in weakness in the joints, loss of flexibility, restricted movement, and a higher risk of injury and pain.

In childhood, most of us have complete range of movement and are able to move around naturally without pain and restriction. As we get older, we start to lose some of this fluidity. We become more sedentary, pick up bad postural habits and, as a result, become stiffer and less flexible.

One of the biggest causes of bad posture lies with your muscles. If you allow them to become tight and restricted (see pages 20–21), they have the power to destroy your postural integrity by causing weakness to your entire body. As they tighten, these muscles start to pull your body out of alignment and disrupt postural balance.

If the natural balance of your posture is compromised, you run a much higher risk of injury and pain. It is, therefore, important to maintain a healthy and posturally stable body regardless of whether you are an active sportsperson or just trying to reclaim the pain-free body that is rightfully yours.

What exactly is good posture and what can you do to achieve it? Well, first you need to understand the forces at play on your body and their knock-on effects.

Like building-blocks, each part of your body must be in good alignment to enable you to stand.

Gravity and structural balance

We are all affected by the impact of gravity, the force that constantly pushes down on us and keeps us with our feet firmly on the ground. Gravity places an astounding 33½ lbs (15 kg) of pressure on every inch of our bodies. Our bodies are designed to resist this force as effectively as possible through the alignment of its various parts to form a strong and stable structure.

Imagine stacking a child's building blocks, one on top of the other. If each block is placed carefully, the structure will be stable, able to bear both its own weight and the weight of gravity. If the building blocks are unevenly stacked, the structure becomes weak, unable to support its own weight, and likely to collapse. Your body works in exactly the same way. It tries to keep everything in line to form a strong, stable, and efficient structure. When all the weight-bearing parts of your body—your own building blocks—are correctly aligned, you are able to oppose the downward force of gravity and remain strong and stable. Good posture is therefore the ability to bear the weight of your body while opposing the constant downward pull of gravity effectively.

When you are structurally balanced, the line of gravity goes straight through the center of your body. As with the building-block tower, you will see that you, too, are made up of various blocks stacked one on top of the other.

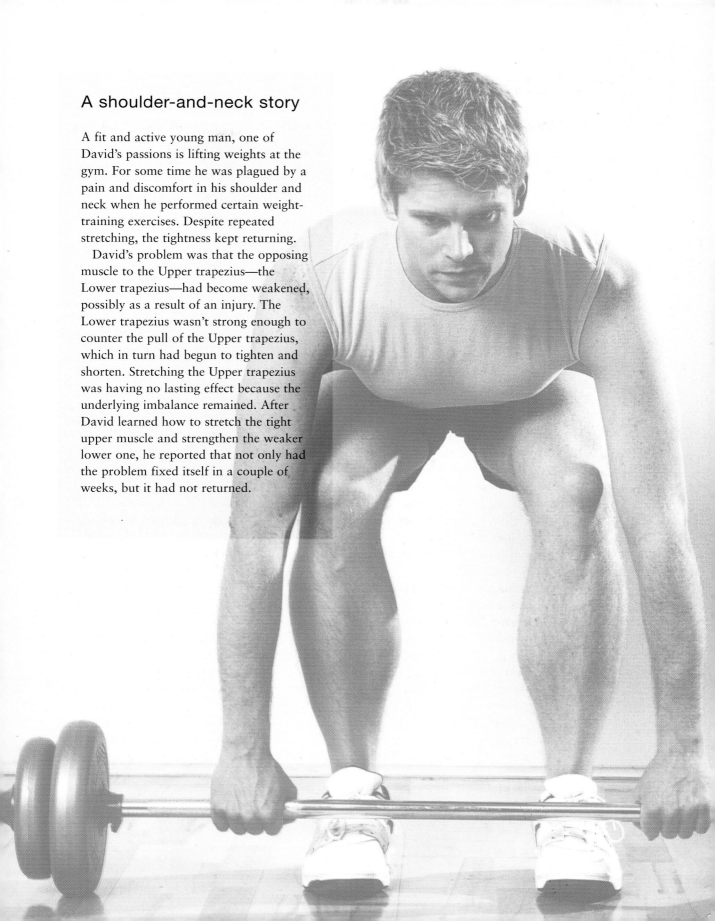

A shoulder-and-neck story

A fit and active young man, one of David's passions is lifting weights at the gym. For some time he was plagued by a pain and discomfort in his shoulder and neck when he performed certain weight-training exercises. Despite repeated stretching, the tightness kept returning.

David's problem was that the opposing muscle to the Upper trapezius—the Lower trapezius—had become weakened, possibly as a result of an injury. The Lower trapezius wasn't strong enough to counter the pull of the Upper trapezius, which in turn had begun to tighten and shorten. Stretching the Upper trapezius was having no lasting effect because the underlying imbalance remained. After David learned how to stretch the tight upper muscle and strengthen the weaker lower one, he reported that not only had the problem fixed itself in a couple of weeks, but it had not returned.

The five body blocks

Your body can be "stacked up" into five supporting blocks: the head and neck (block 1); the shoulders, chest, and upper back (block 2); the lower back and hips (block 3); the upper legs and knees (block 4); the lower legs and feet (block 5). Each of these blocks must be structurally strong for you to have postural stability.

At the heart of each block, the bones and joints sustain the most weight. If your body is positioned correctly, the center of each block will line up from the front, the back, and the side.

The path of gravity

Looking at your body from the front and back (see pictures opposite), the primary supporting structure is the spine, and, as long as the line of gravity passes through it, your body will be strong and balanced. The line of gravity passes directly through the head, the nasal septum, and straight down the bones of the neck (cervicals) in block 1. As you continue down, the line courses through the center of the breastbone and the upper and middle bones of the spine (thoracic vertebrae) in block 2. Then, it passes centrally through the bones in the lower back (lumbar vertebrae) and the pelvis through the middle of the pubic bone, the sacrum, and the coccyx at the rear in block 3.

From the front and back, blocks 4 and 5 are less important to your posture because the gravity line does not actually penetrate any solid part once it leaves the body via the bottom of the pelvis. What is important is for both legs to be evenly spaced either side of the gravity line.

When you view your body from the side, your ears, shoulders, hips, knees, and ankles should all follow a straight vertical line (see picture far right). The gravity line starts at the top of the head, then passes through the opening of the ear (auditory miatus), continuing down through the

bones in your neck in block 1. The weight of your head, which makes up about one-tenth of your total weight, is supported by the cervicals, the bones in your neck connecting to your spine. As the line continues traveling down, it should go through the shoulder joint in block 2. Then, the gravity line comes down through the strongest and most stable portion of your lower spine. As it leaves your backbone, the line of gravity crosses the midpoint of your hip joint in block 3. You can see from the position of the gravity line that the long bone in your thigh (femur) and the knee joint are the major weight bearers in block 4. Finally, the gravity line passes through your shinbone (tibia) and comes to rest just in front of your anklebone (external maliolus) in block 5.

If your body is centered with all the blocks in their correct positions, your body will work with and not against you, your bones will provide the necessary support, and your muscles will be free to generate smooth, unhindered movement. A stronger, more resilient body will improve your health levels, allow for greater mobility, and greatly reduce the likelihood of pain and injury.

Adapting to bad posture

Unfortunately, due to bad postural habits, physical imbalances, and inflexibility brought on by both the way we live our lives and also through injury, many of us no longer oppose the dynamic force of gravity as efficiently as our bodies were designed to do. When your posture is compromised, your inability to support your

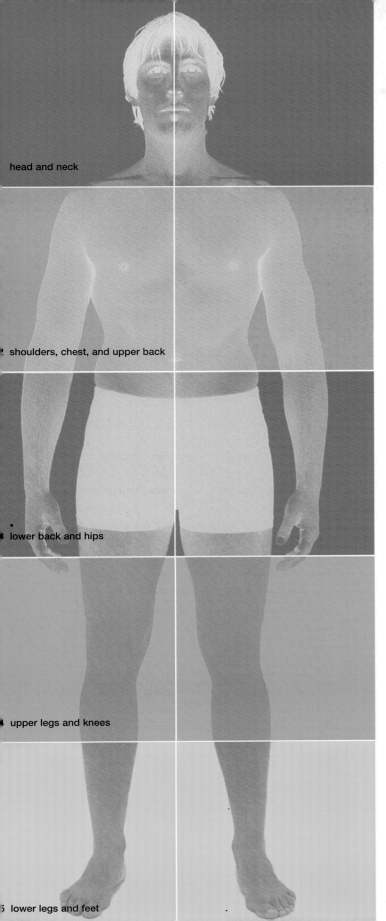

head and neck

shoulders, chest, and upper back

lower back and hips

upper legs and knees

lower legs and feet

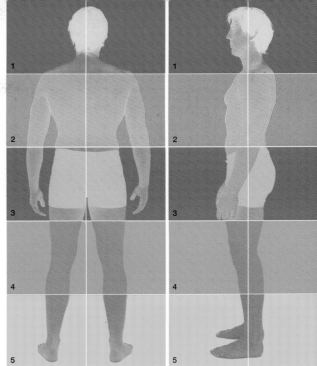

1
2
3
4
5

With optimal posture, the line of gravity runs through the center of each block, from the front, the back, and the side.

own body weight and resist gravity competently can have devastating effects. As your body moves out of alignment, a whole series of adaptations take place.

An unstable core

Your pelvis forms the basis and foundation of your overall postural stability. If it is not aligned and structurally secure, the rest of your body won't be either. Anatomically, the "core" of your body is at the level of your sacrum, the flat triangular bone at the base of your spine. From the front, it is located about 2 inches (5 cm) below your navel in the pelvic area. If your pelvis, for example, is tilted forward, a postural knock-on effect will reverberate through your whole body. Starting at the hips and working down, let's examine the repercussions from an incorrect forward rotation of the pelvis.

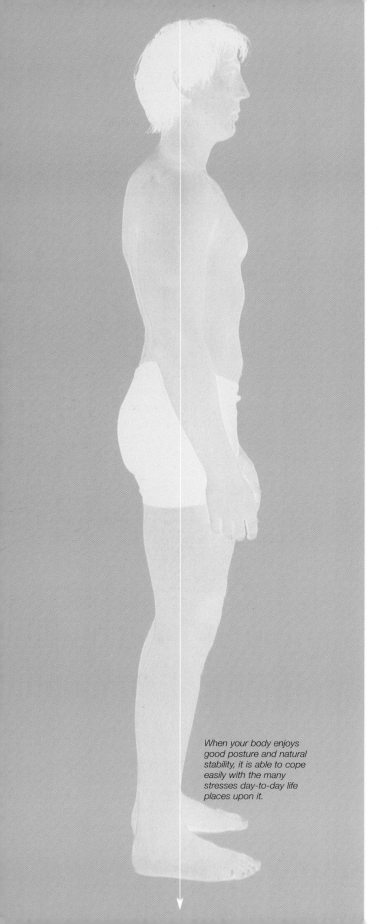

When your body enjoys good posture and natural stability, it is able to cope easily with the many stresses day-to-day life places upon it.

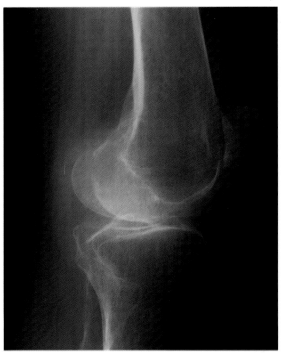

Locked-back knees can cause the ligaments and cartilage to become overstressed and start to deteriorate.

Locked-back knees

When you stand up naturally, your knees should have a slight bend to them and not be completely locked back. Check yourself and observe how friends and colleagues are standing. You will find that many of them have their knees in locked mode, one of the telltale signs that there is a detrimental forward rotation of the pelvis.

Locked-back knees cause the leg bones to be pushed back and they start to lose their efficiency at holding you up. Instead, the muscles at the front of your thighs are forced to act as primary weight-bearing supports. The longer you are in this position, the tighter the muscles get and the more tension they hold. This backward pressure can cause the knee joints to become weakened and misaligned.

As a result of locked-back knees, the bones of the lower legs (the tibia and fibula) come to be positioned behind the gravity line, once again

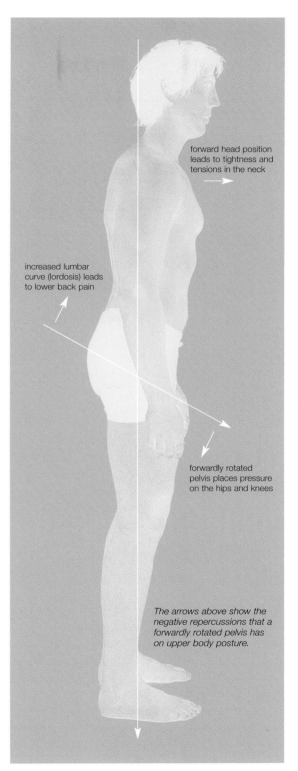

forward head position leads to tightness and tensions in the neck

increased lumbar curve (lordosis) leads to lower back pain

forwardly rotated pelvis places pressure on the hips and knees

The arrows above show the negative repercussions that a forwardly rotated pelvis has on upper body posture.

forcing the soft tissues of the legs (muscles, tendons, and ligaments) to become tight and restricted in order to support your body weight.

A forward tilt

While everything below a rotated pelvis is pulled back, everything above it is pushed forward. The bones in the lower back are edged forward. Just as with the legs, the muscles and ligaments of the lower back are now forced to act as weight bearers. Muscle tightness, combined with the forward position, causes compression to the joints and discs, leading to lower-back problems.

The supporting bones of the neck are also pulled forward, and the muscles, tendons, and ligaments at the back of the neck have to adapt to support the weight of your head. This can lead to compression, restriction, and pain. As your shoulders are pulled forward, they become rounded and hunched, and this not only leads to problems in the shoulders but can contribute to respiratory difficulties.

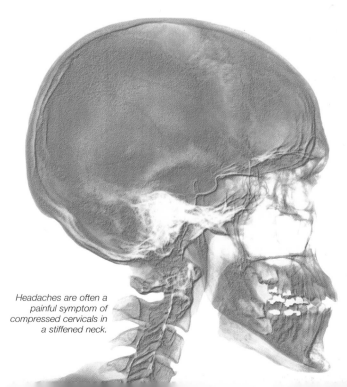

Headaches are often a painful symptom of compressed cervicals in a stiffened neck.

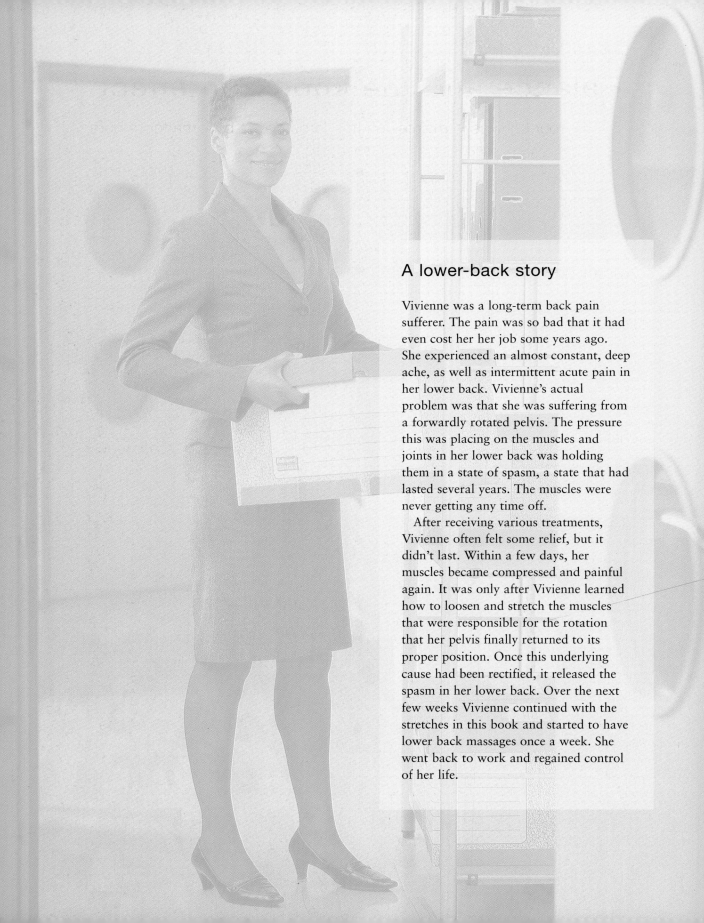

A lower-back story

Vivienne was a long-term back pain sufferer. The pain was so bad that it had even cost her her job some years ago. She experienced an almost constant, deep ache, as well as intermittent acute pain in her lower back. Vivienne's actual problem was that she was suffering from a forwardly rotated pelvis. The pressure this was placing on the muscles and joints in her lower back was holding them in a state of spasm, a state that had lasted several years. The muscles were never getting any time off.

After receiving various treatments, Vivienne often felt some relief, but it didn't last. Within a few days, her muscles became compressed and painful again. It was only after Vivienne learned how to loosen and stretch the muscles that were responsible for the rotation that her pelvis finally returned to its proper position. Once this underlying cause had been rectified, it released the spasm in her lower back. Over the next few weeks Vivienne continued with the stretches in this book and started to have lower back massages once a week. She went back to work and regained control of her life.

Balance and the knock-on effect

Your balance is maintained to a large extent by a matter of pure reflex. You don't have to think about it, it just happens. When your head is level and your eyes and ears are on an even plane, it is easy for your body to maintain its balance, but tilting your head makes keeping your balance much more difficult.

Tilting upsets the delicate workings of your inner ear, which contains a motion-sensing mechanism called the vestibular system. This consists of three semicircular canals and two tiny organs (the saccule and the utricle) that detect any motion of your head. When you move your head, fluid within the vestibular system triggers nerve impulses that tell your brain about the movement. Acting on this information, your brain controls your muscles to help you keep your balance.

The righting reflex

The ancient, biologically programmed part of your brain knows that without the ability to maintain your balance you cannot run from danger, hunt for food, or perform the many varied functions necessary for your survival. Therefore, your body has been brilliantly equipped to ensure that you are properly balanced at all times. It does this with a hardwired "righting reflex" specifically designed to make sure that your eyes and ears stay level.

Try this experiment for yourself. Tilt your head to one side and try to walk along in a straight line. You will find that it is quite difficult and it takes some effort to stop yourself from veering off to one side. If you were to keep walking with your head tilted you would soon start to feel dizzy and would most likely fall down. This is why your body places so much emphasis on balance. If you cannot maintain it, you become extremely vulnerable.

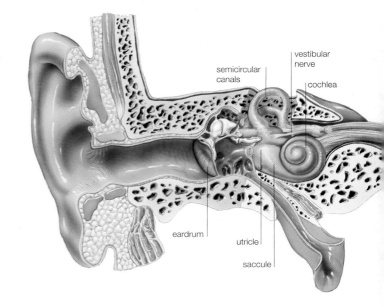

The vestibular system (the utricle, saccule, and semicircular canals) within your inner ear helps you to maintain your balance. When you move your head, fluid within the system moves and pulls on sensory hairs that trigger signals in the vestibular nerve.

If your posture becomes distorted, whether through bad postural habits or through injury, your righting reflex will bring into play a series of postural adaptations and adjustments that will twist, turn, buckle, and distort your body. This cataclysmic knock-on effect spreads throughout your body as it attempts to cancel out the unwanted original distortion and return your eyes and ears to an even plane and restore optimum balance.

The effect of distortions

In the case of a forwardly rotated pelvis, for example, your upper body is forced into a forward-leaning position. As you can see in the first diagram on the right, this moves your body away from the ideal path of gravity (see page 20) as the weight of your chest, shoulders, and head moves forward. This then forces your body to make a series of adjustments (the knock-on effect) to compensate for the distortion.

Your body will not allow you to simply lean forward as this could compromise both your balance and stability. Instead, it adjusts itself to keep your eyes and ears level, as you can see from the second diagram. The eyes are now level, but unfortunately, your body has compensated for the original distortion by contracting the muscles in your neck to lift your head up. This will lead to tightness, restriction, and, in all probability, a literal pain in the neck.

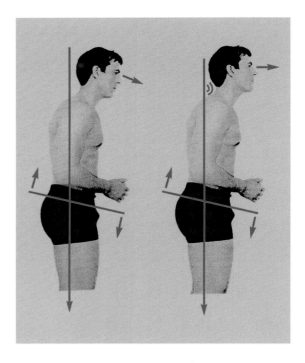

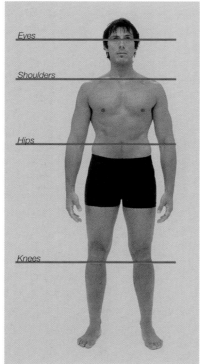

Eyes

Shoulders

Hips

Knees

The horizontal plane

As well as keeping your eyes level, your body also wants to keep your back as straight as possible. It is constantly trying to keep you as upright and balanced as it possibly can. Looking from the front, as in the diagram on the left, your eyes, ears, shoulders, and hips should all be lined up horizontally to ensure optimum biomechanical output. The more posturally distorted you become, the greater will be the negative effect on your biomechanics.

As a result of the way you are constructed, if either your pelvis or your shoulders move off of the horizontal plane, it becomes impossible for you to maintain a healthy, straight spine. This not only has a major effect on your physical structure, it also hinders the internal workings of your body. And if your hips tilt to one side and become uneven, your spine and therefore your whole body will also tilt. Your body will then seek to straighten your spine once again to keep your eyes level.

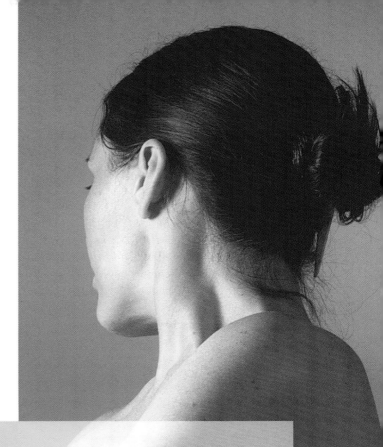

Twisting

Another powerful movement pattern is the physical force of torque (twisting). If, for example, your right shoulder is being pushed forward and your left shoulder is being pulled backward, your spine starts to rotate. This generates an huge amount of compression and force on the area between these two points.

Think about the action of wringing out a towel. As you twist both ends in different directions, it doesn't take much strength for you to really squeeze the section of the towel between your hands. If your shoulders are twisting one way and your hips are twisting in the opposite direction, think about the amount of pressure you are placing on your spine. Of all the postural and biomechanical distortions that your body can have, twisting is the most devastating. It is responsible for much of the tearing, rupturing, and herniation of discs in the spine.

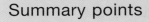

Summary points

- The body is a marvellous system of pulleys and levers: bones, joints, ligaments, muscles, and tendons. Their structures and interaction strengthen the body's framework and make movement, coordination, and agility possible.

- Muscles work in pairs. Every time you make a movement there is an opposing muscle that allows you to make a counter movement.

- A bone or joint stays correctly aligned only if the amount of pull (muscle tone) placed on it by each set of opposing muscles is equal in force. An imbalance in this dynamic can cause the body to deviate from its natural position.

Shorter, tighter muscles can destroy your postural integrity.

- One misalignment of the body can cause a knock-on effect to other parts. These misalignments can cause muscles to get tighter and tenser, joints to become weakened and stressed, and connective tissue to break down, leading to discomfort and pain.

- Twisting and torque in the body is responsible for much of the tearing, rupturing, or herniation of spinal discs.

- Maintaining postural integrity and preventing pain is a matter of balance between pairs of muscles.

Pain: friend or foe?

More often than not, pain is seen as an unwelcome and negative intrusion to be eradicated at all costs. However, there has been a marked shift in perception. Pain should no longer be seen as a "villain," but more as a hard-working messenger, relaying crucial information to which we must listen.

Whatever your personal experience of pain, be it a recent injury, a long-term problem, or simply the unavoidable knocks, bumps, and scrapes of day-to-day living, you will no doubt be familiar with how disruptive it can be to the quality of your life. In order to understand how to relieve pain effectively, you must first understand what it is, what causes it, what it means, how it affects your body, and how to deal with it.

The nervous system

The nervous system acts as the hard wiring for your body and is made up of two parts: part one consists of your brain and spinal cord; part two is made up of the immense network of nerves that cover and pass through every part of your body. The nerves in your body are arranged in much the same way as the branches of a tree. From your spinal cord come thick nerves, which continually divide and spread out to reach every part of your body. This amazing network allows you, with the help of various sensors, to feel all the sensations in and around you, including pain.

The body's sensors

You have three main types of sensor that pick up and send information to your brain. Exteroceptors tell you about the external environment, detecting touch and temperature sensations (as well as the specialized senses of sight, smell, and hearing); proprioceptors, found in joints and tendons, monitor changes in position and movement; and enteroceptors,

found in the digestive, respiratory, cardiovascular, urinary, and reproductive systems, that pick up sensations such as hunger and thirst. When activated, these sensors send an electrical impulse along your nerves, into your spinal cord and to your brain, which interprets them and makes the appropriate response.

Movement impulses

However, this is not the only function of the nervous system. Each nerve is like a telephone wire through which messages and information can be sent and received. In the same way that you can have a two-way conversation on the telephone, the various parts of your body can send messages to your brain and the brain can send signals to the appropriate parts of your body. For example, to pick up a pen, your brain sends an electrical signal into the muscles of your fingers and hand, making them contract. These contractions move the individual bones in your fingers and hand, and you pick up the pen.

This conversation between your body and brain happens 24 hours a day and, when everything's running smoothly, you feel calm and comfortable. But not all conversations go well and some can cause you stress or anger. Similarly, when the calm, rhythmical impulses from your nerves are replaced by strong, rapid signals, this is often interpreted by your brain as pain.

Once the workings of pain are clear, you will realize what an ally it really can be.

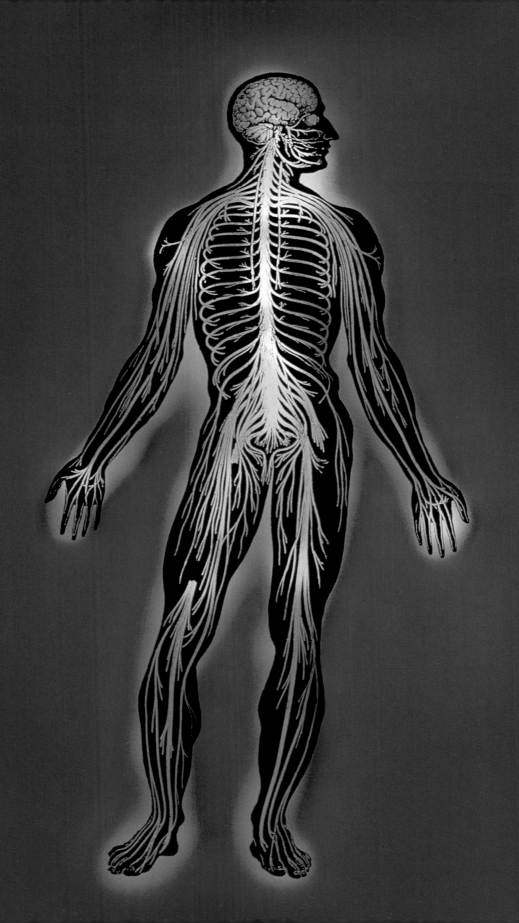

What is pain?

Pain is a signal, an agitated electrical impulse that is sent along your nerves and into your brain. If you tear a muscle or break a bone, it is not the muscle or bone that generates the pain but the nerves that surround and permeate it. For example, a person who is paralyzed, and has lost the use of his or her legs, cannot feel any pain in these limbs even though they still consist of living and growing muscles, ligaments, and bones. The brain can send the signals, but because the nervous system has been damaged, the muscles no longer receive them, just as the receptor signals from the nerves in the legs no longer reach the brain.

An early warning system

The key thing about pain is that it can help prevent serious injury by acting as an early warning system. Pain is simply your body's way of saying there is something wrong. The sensible thing to do is to take heed of this warning and to fix the underlying problem.

We live in a society that supports the widespread advertising and endorsement of painkillers, and pharmaceutical companies seek to convince us that pain itself is what needs to be eradicated. Numbing the pain has become the socially acceptable thing to do. As soon as we get the slightest pain we immediately reach for the painkillers and analgesic rubs. Admittedly, in some cases, painkillers are the most effective way of dealing with the sensation of pain, but they should be used diligently and only when there is really no other available alternative.

Causes of pain

Many things can cause the nerve impulses to fire more rapidly and so create the sensation of pain. Burning yourself, cutting yourself, and tearing muscle or connective tissue all cause enough negative sensory input for your nervous system to become highly agitated.

Trapped nerves

However, the most common cause of pain is nerve entrapment. This occurs when the nerves that run through the muscles become confined and squeezed. When a muscle gets too tight, it can squeeze the nerves inside it. This then agitates these nerves, causing them to send out stronger and quicker impulses to the brain. As the nerves continue to "fire" more rapidly, the increase in electrical impulses being sent into your brain is registered as pain.

For a clearer demonstration of how this works, place the

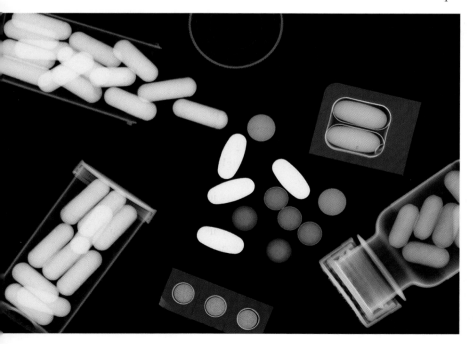

As a society, we are now in the bad habit of relying on all manner of pills and potions to help us deal with our everyday aches and pains.

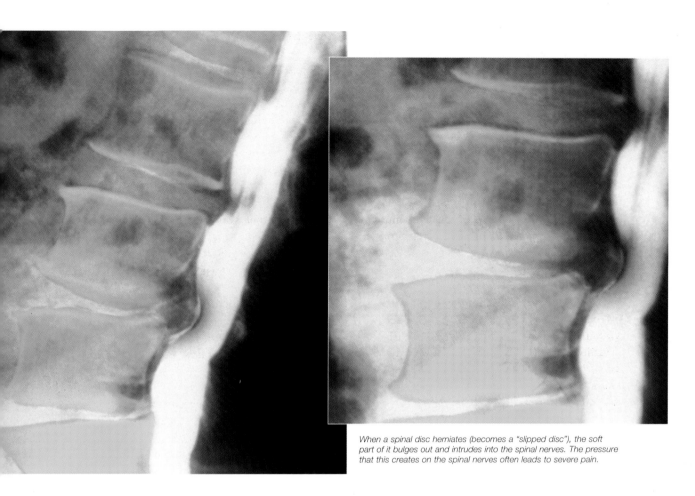

When a spinal disc herniates (becomes a "slipped disc"), the soft part of it bulges out and intrudes into the spinal nerves. The pressure that this creates on the spinal nerves often leads to severe pain.

index finger of your right hand on your left palm. Gently close your left hand around your right finger. Your left hand represents the muscle and your right index finger represents a nerve. When you squeeze your left hand you will feel the pressure on your right finger increase—squeeze harder still and the pressure increases. In other words the more the muscle is tightened, the more pressure is placed on the nerve.

Compressed nerves

Pain also may be triggered by bones pushing down on the nerves or by the cartilage between the bones moving and pressing down on the nerves. This is called nerve compression, and anyone who has ever suffered from a "slipped disc" has fallen victim to this effect. In such cases, the cartilage disc between the bones of the spine bulges out and puts pressure on the nerve root, causing pain and discomfort.

We can see from this that tight, restricted muscles can be responsible for much of the pain we experience. So what makes a muscle tight? As well as being able to consciously contract your muscles they can also be shortened by an automatic reflex action. This is all part of your body's self-defense system.

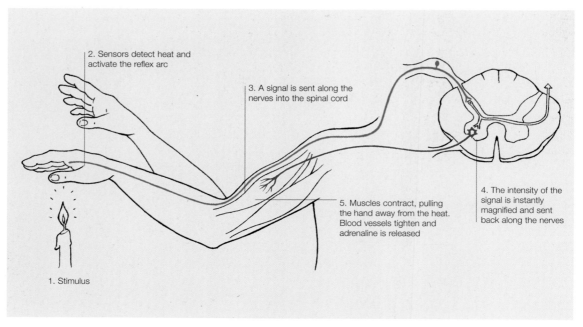

2. Sensors detect heat and activate the reflex arc

3. A signal is sent along the nerves into the spinal cord

4. The intensity of the signal is instantly magnified and sent back along the nerves

5. Muscles contract, pulling the hand away from the heat. Blood vessels tighten and adrenaline is released

1. Stimulus

The body's protective reflex action in motion. This example shows how the reflex arc makes you automatically pull your hand away from the heat of a candle flame.

The reflex arc

If you have ever burned yourself in the kitchen or accidentally splashed your hands with scalding water, you will know that the immediate reaction is to pull your hand quickly away from the source of heat. You don't even have to think about it, you just do it. This is because it is a protective reflex that is so hardwired into your nervous system that it doesn't require the intervention of your brain. Even the small amount of time it would take you to consciously realize that something was too hot and to then move your hand away may still not be quick enough to stop serious damage from occurring. For this reason, as soon as the excessive heat is sensed, a signal is sent along your nerves into your spinal cord, where the intensity of this signal is immediately magnified and sent back down the nerves into the muscles of your arm and hand telling them to contract. This automatic reaction, called a reflex arc, takes place in a fraction of a second. The result is

that your hand is pulled away from the heat source and removed from danger in the fastest time possible.

This reflex not only protects you from heat, it is a kind of general safety mechanism and is the way your body protects itself from all sudden and dangerous physical forces placed upon it. Let's take another example. If you overstretch your shoulder, perhaps during a fall or while participating in sports, this reflex action is activated to help save your joint. As your shoulder is forced beyond its normal range of motion, the joint starts to be pulled open. The further the joint is stretched, the more unstable it becomes, and the greater the risk of serious damage. The sensors in the ligaments that hold the joint together register this rapid and dangerous change. They immediately send a danger signal into the spinal cord, which activates the reflex safety mechanism. This reflex, in turn, causes the muscles around the joint to shorten dramatically and so pull the joint back together. In addition, neighboring blood vessels tighten to restrict blood flow in the area and, therefore, limit any internal bleeding from possibly torn tissues. The kidneys also release adrenaline to help you deal with the situation. All these responses happen automatically and in a fraction of a second. Although you may end up with sore and possibly slightly strained muscles around your shoulder for a few days, without the reflex arc you may have suffered serious or permanent damage to the joint.

The relevance of this reflex arc and its implications in the realm of pain will become clearer once another vital piece of the pain puzzle is in place—trigger points.

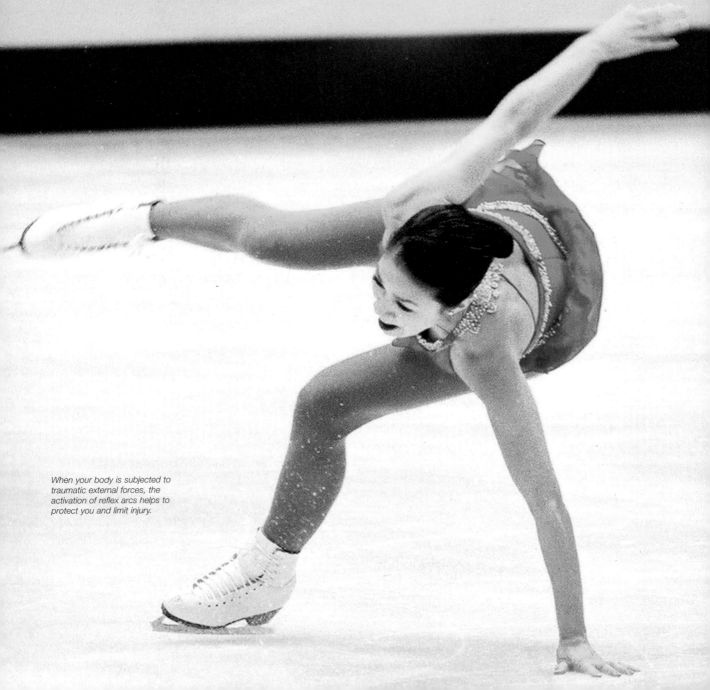

When your body is subjected to traumatic external forces, the activation of reflex arcs helps to protect you and limit injury.

Trigger points

Whenever your body sustains some kind of damage, the affected area almost invariably becomes painful or sore. As we have already seen, pain and discomfort are the result of excess stress placed on the nerves, which then send stronger, more rapid impulses into the brain. The cause of such stress can come from several sources. When you have a light injury, the nerves can be agitated due to the protective tightening of the surrounding muscles. With more serious injuries, pain is caused by the actual tearing of the tissues and the subsequent rupturing of some of the tiny nerves that pass through them.

Sometimes the tenderness and pain that you feel can be a warning that, although not injured, the muscle itself is becoming too tight and restricted. As flexibility is lost and the muscle becomes constricted, the nerves running through the muscle will become more compressed, just as in the finger squeezing demonstration on page 31. However, there is another pain mechanism that is vitally important to maintaining a healthy, pain-free body.

Pain referral

Soreness or pain can often be the result of trigger points. These are very localized areas of damage that not only feel sore and painful to the touch, but also have a unique ability to send sensations of pain and discomfort to other parts of the body via the nervous system. As well as pain, these sensations can include numbness, heat, cold, "pins and needles," and a feeling of heaviness. For example, when a trigger point is formed in the infraspinatus muscle (at the back of your shoulder), it not only causes localized pain but also has the ability to refer pain to the side of the shoulder and down the arm. If you do feel pain in your arm but don't know that the pain is originating in the infraspinatus muscle, no matter how much you treat your arm, the problem will remain until the trigger point in the muscle itself has been released.

As you can see, trigger points can be responsible for many seemingly inexplicable aches and pains. How often do you hear somebody saying "My back hurts, but I don't remember doing anything to it?" This could be the result of a trigger point.

Causes of trigger points

Whenever a muscle becomes tight or overstressed in some way, trigger points can form. They may be the result of a direct injury or they may have been caused by continual stress being placed on the muscle from persistent overuse and strain. Trigger points send out very strong and prolonged nerve impulses. Such a sustained input can have a potentially upsetting and distressing effect on the body's normal safety reflex mechanism. Although found mainly in muscles, trigger points can also appear in other areas of the body, such as tendons, ligaments, and other connective tissue.

As we have already seen, your body normally responds to high levels of impulses by activating the reflex arc. Trigger points, on the other hand, create a whole different ball game. When the signals entering the spinal cord are very strong and sustained, the safety mechanism can start to work against you, resulting in chronic pain. This is how it works.

Chronic pain

When a trigger point "fires," the sensors in the body detect these agitated impulses and the reflex arc is activated. But a trigger point emits constant, sustained impulses, so even after the reflex arc has been activated the trigger point continues to "fire" away, activating the reflex arc again and again. Indeed, one of the most disruptive qualities of trigger points is their ability not only to produce pain, but also to interfere with the body's natural reflex arcs.

The resulting contractions of the muscles and blood vessels in the area actually compound the problem. As the muscles tighten, more stress is placed on the trigger point. The trigger point then sends stronger impulses into the spinal cord, which causes the muscles to get even tighter, which causes the trigger point to send even stronger impulses, and so on. Once this negative, self-perpetuating situation is in place, the cycle of pain and discomfort can last for years and years, or until the trigger point is deactivated.

Trigger points are always found in tight, constricted muscles. If you find an area that "triggers" sensations in another part of the body when you press into it, then your body is telling you that that particular muscle is already overloaded. If the muscle is left untreated, you could eventually find yourself with chronic pain, dysfunction, or restriction. The remaining pain may not even be the spot where the trigger point originated, but the place to which the pain is radiating. This causes inexplicable pains in parts of your body that you don't ever remember hurting or straining. This on its own should be an incentive, if ever there was one, for keeping your muscles flexible and healthy.

The pain coming from a trigger point located in one part of the body may be felt as sensations in a completely different area.

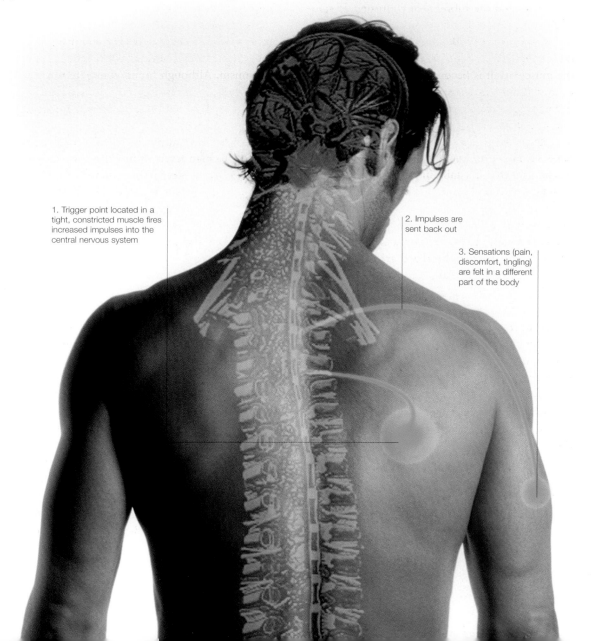

1. Trigger point located in a tight, constricted muscle fires increased impulses into the central nervous system

2. Impulses are sent back out

3. Sensations (pain, discomfort, tingling) are felt in a different part of the body

Relieving pain

Whether you are suffering from a recent injury or a more long-term problem, pain and discomfort can have a detrimental effect on your physical performance and your ability to enjoy life to the full. If this is the case for you, easing pain will no doubt be high on your list of priorities.

There are two possible solutions for eliminating the sensation of pain: blocking out the signal or removing its cause.

Blocking the signal

The easiest, and by far the most common, way to block pain is to use painkillers and analgesics. These do not make the pain and its cause go away, painkillers simply suppress our ability to feel it. Taking again the example of someone who is paralyzed, that person still has all the physical elements needed to produce pain but because of the injury to their spinal cord, which carries the pain signal, the message does not make it to the brain. When you take painkillers, the same thing happens. The signal is blocked from entering your brain, only this time it is done chemically. The cause of the pain is still there, the pain signals are still being sent from the injured area, you just don't feel them any more.

One of the main problems with this approach to pain relief is that pain often acts as a form of protection against greater damage and trauma. It should be fairly obvious that if you have hurt a part of your body, the more you use it, the greater the risk of making the injury worse. Imagine twisting your ankle and then deciding to go for a jog. The already strained and weakened ligaments of your ankle would not, in all likelihood, be strong or stable enough to withstand the added movement and stress of jogging. Before you knew it, you would have serious pain and ligament damage. To stop this

from happening your body tries to ensure that you do not go for that jog, that you instead keep the ankle still and refrain from putting extra stress on it. And how does it do this? Simple: by creating pain.

Pain is a major incentive to keep an injured area still, so giving it time to heal. It's simple: you move, it hurts; you keep still, the pain stops, so you keep still. If you remove pain by blocking the signal, keep in mind that the cause of pain still exists and that movement puts you at risk of making the injury worse.

Illustrating the function of pain

It can be useful to think of pain as a warning light, pre-empting injury and mechanical dysfunction. Let's use a familiar example to illustrate this.

Cars are fitted with several warning mechanisms, one of which is the oil-pressure light. Of course, it is very important for the running of your car that it has sufficient oil. If the car runs out of oil or if, for some reason, the oil is not flowing smoothly, there is nothing to lubricate the moving parts of the engine. This causes friction and soon this friction, coupled with the intense heat that it generates, causes the moving parts of the car to seize up. The car breaks down and the engine is ruined. To prevent such mechanical damage, your car is fitted with an oil-pressure warning light. When the oil level in the car starts to drop down to a dangerous level, the light on the dashboard comes on. Your

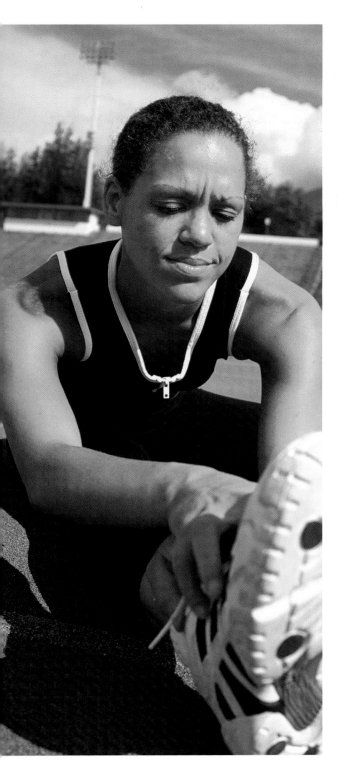

The FIRST approach

1 The warning light comes on.

2 You recognize that it is a warning and understand that the light coming on is not the problem in itself, but that it is alerting you to a problem with the oil pressure.

3 You take action to rectify the cause, perhaps by putting more oil in the car or by checking the oil pump.

4 Once you have solved the problem the light goes off.

The SECOND approach

1 The warning light comes on.

2 You disconnect the wires leading to the warning light

3 The warning light is no longer illuminated so you believe the problem has been solved.

objective in such a situation is to get the warning light to switch off. The sequence of events to achieve this is very simple and straightforward. Even someone with no mechanical knowledge can see that the second approach is not the best approach. Although the light has gone off, the underlying cause has not gone away. If the car continues to be driven it will break down.

Pain is your "warning light." It is telling you that somewhere in your body excess pressure is being applied to the nerves and overstimulating them. The correct course of action is to locate the cause and eliminate it. The pain signals will then stop. When you block the signal chemically by taking painkillers, it's as if you are disconnecting your "warning light."

When you feel pain, it is your body's way of warning you of a problem.

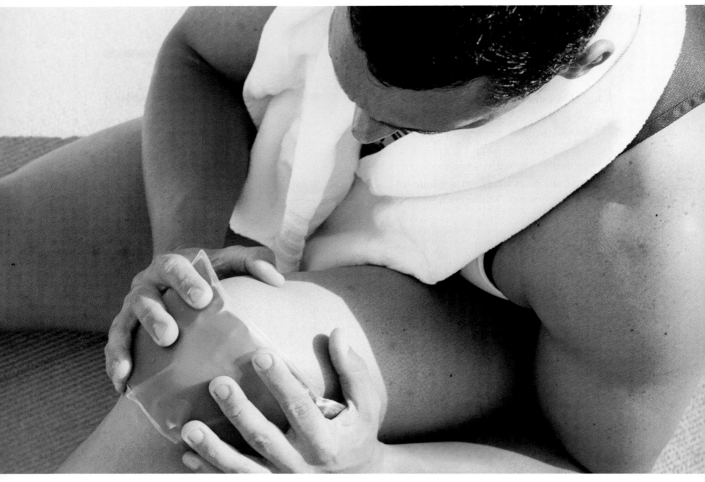

Hot packs increase blood flow so they are ideal for treating chronic muscular aches. Cold packs decrease blood flow so they are better suited to treating acute swellings.

Removing the cause

The second way to deal with pain is to remove the cause. It doesn't take a rocket scientist to realize that this is the most preferable way by far. Since we already know the mechanics of pain and what causes it, we can use this information to deal with it. Simply follow the easy three-step approach: irrigate – eradicate – elongate.

Step 1: Irrigate

This means to increase the supply of blood to the injured area. Blood can be thought of as your body's conveyer belt, carrying nutrients and oxygen, which it receives via the lungs each time you inhale. The oxygen, which your body converts into energy, allows each of your individual cells to function properly. Like any energy-producing process, this procedure also creates waste products, in this case carbon dioxide and various acids. These enter the blood stream and are removed from it when you exhale, and the whole process starts again with the next breath. The greater the amount of blood you can get to a particular area, the more oxygen and nutrients that area receives, and the better its ability to remove any waste products.

It is extremely important for the health of your muscles, and of every cell in your body, that they receive an adequate blood supply. If an area is injured or damaged, this becomes even more important. Just imagine what would happen to you if you couldn't get all the food and water you needed and were also unable to eliminate your body's waste products adequately—you would soon start feeling ill. Now imagine that you were already ill before this situation started—you would most likely get a whole lot worse, a whole lot quicker. The same applies to muscles and other structures in your body. The more blood that flows in and around the damaged area, the quicker it will heal. It is also worth noting that some of the waste products produced in the energy creation process, can in themselves cause irritation to the nerves and soreness in the muscles if they are not removed.

There are several very effective ways to increase blood supply to the affected area, but one of the best and easiest is massage. For a guide to the best way to massage for pain relief, see the box on the right. Another simple way to increase blood supply to an area is the use of heat. This works very well when used in conjunction with massage. After you have massaged the area, a heat pack or even a hot water bottle can be placed on it. The heat dilates the capillaries, the small blood vessels that surround the muscles. As they expand, more blood is able to pass through them. There are also many different type of heat rubs and sprays available, which have the same effect. Professional therapists often use ultrasound, which has been shown to help promote blood flow to an injured area. Ultrasound uses high-frequency sound waves to produce heat and movement deep in muscles, ligaments, and tendons.

Caution: although it is necessary to increase blood flow in order to heal an injured area this should not be done immediately following a bad injury. One of the reasons for this is that if any

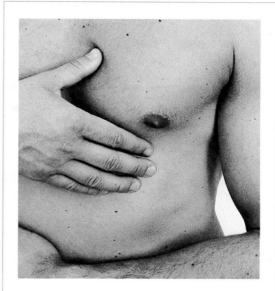

MASSAGE FOR PAIN RELIEF
Using your thumb or your index and middle fingers, massage and gently knead the affected area in long, even strokes. Work across the area in 1/2 to 1-inch (1 to 2.5-cm) wide strips. Knead each strip 8–10 times before moving across to the next strip. Repeat until you have covered the whole area. Although this massage shouldn't cause pain, a mild sense of discomfort is acceptable. You can repeat this procedure two to three times at each treatment. Treat the area once or twice a day.

of the muscles or other tissues were torn in the injury, there could well be internal bleeding. If this is the case, pushing even more blood into the damaged area will increase the blood loss. Also, the heat generated by the increased blood flow can make any swelling much worse and interfere with the body's natural healing process. See the box on page 40 for more information on first aid for injuries.

If the pain and swelling are severe, consult a doctor. You don't have to do it all yourself. An important part of true independence is the ability to make informed choices. This often involves choosing the best person for the job.

FIRST AID FOR STRAINS AND SPRAINS

The general guidelines to follow for the first
two to three days after a severe injury are represented by
the acronym RICE, which stands for Rest, Ice, Compress,
and Elevate.

Rest: Avoid moving or stressing the injured area. If the
injury is located on your feet, ankles, or legs, stay off your
feet as much as possible.

Ice: Apply an ice pack or cold compress (a bag of frozen
peas works well) to the injured area for about 10 minutes.
Repeat regularly throughout the day, allowing at least two
hours between each application, but never put an ice pack
directly on the skin. Use a thin towel as a barrier.

Compress: Firmly bandage or strap the injured area, but
not so tight that you restrict the blood supply. Compression
helps minimize swelling and provides further support to the
injured area by helping to limit movement.

Elevate: Wherever possible, try to keep the injured area
raised above the level of your heart. The best position for
this is lying down with the injured area propped up to the
appropriate level using pillows or cushions. Elevation helps
reduce swelling and inflammation; this relieves the pain and
speeds up the healing process.

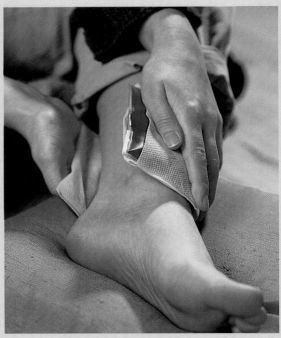

*Applying ice to an acute injury helps to alleviate immediate pain
and reduces swelling.*

Step 2: Eradicate

If you massage an area and it is sore then it is a
sign that the area is suffering from a lack of
circulation (ischemia). If, however, you find that
a particular spot "triggers" a sensation
somewhere other than where you are pressing,
then you've found a trigger point. If there are
any trigger points present in an injured area, they
need to be eliminated. A muscle cannot maintain
its normal flexibility if it contains a trigger point.

Again, there are several ways you can
eradicate trigger points, including freezing the
area and acupuncture. But one of the easiest and
most effective ways to deal with trigger points is
through simple, direct pressure. This makes it
very easy for you to treat trigger points yourself,
or, if you can't reach the exact spot, to get
someone else to press it for you.

Without getting too technical, the way it
works is like this. As you already know, if

something hurts or is causing you discomfort, the
nerves are already being overstimulated. Adding
physical pressure to the damaged area increases
this stimulation further, causing the nerves to
"fire" even more rapidly. However, when you
continue to apply pressure to a trigger point,
after an initial increase, the overall rate of
stimulation begins to drop.

For example, let's say that while massaging
(irrigating) a muscle in your arm you located a
trigger point. Suppose this trigger point was
stimulating the nerves at a rate of six times more
than normal. If direct pressure were applied to
the trigger point, the stimulation of the area
would increase initially to eight times greater
than normal. The result would be that pain
would increase and you would feel sensations
radiating to other parts of the body. After about
8 to 12 seconds, the pain and referred sensations
would start to reduce. This is the point at which

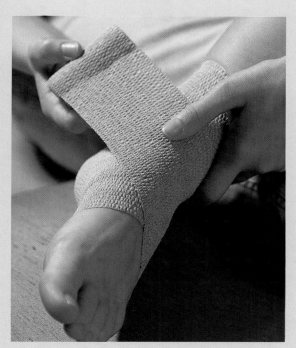

If you feel a strong throbbing when compressing an injured area, remove the bandage and reapply it a little looser.

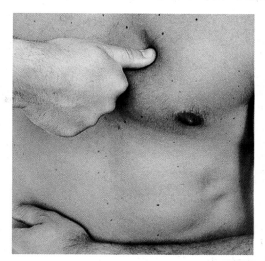

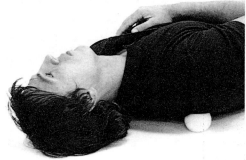

you should stop pressing. Amazingly, the trigger point would now be stimulating your nervous system at a rate of only four times greater than normal. If you repeated the process a few minutes later, the trigger point would initially increase from firing at a rate four times greater than normal (the new starting point) to six times greater than normal. Stopping after 8 to 12 seconds of sustained, even pressure, would cause the firing rate to drop again to only two times greater than normal. Each time pressure is applied like this the amount of stimulation decreases. After the third time the nervous system is "firing" at its normal rate once more. The trigger point has now been deactivated.

Turn to Part Three for a detailed look at the potential pain referral zones caused by trigger points in each muscle.

TREATING TRIGGER POINTS

Caution: do not push too hard when pressing into a trigger point. A moderate pressure of about 10 lbs (4.5 kg) should be enough. You can practice how hard you should push by pushing your thumb down on a set of scales. Remember, the body likes calm, steady impulses. If you dig your thumb into the trigger point, this can upset things and lead to the area becoming tighter.

Trigger points in hard-to-reach places can be released by using a tennis ball or similar. Place the ball on the floor—not a bed as this will be too soft. Sit or lie with the ball underneath your affected muscles. Slowly move around to locate tender areas and trigger points. If you find a trigger point simply relax, allowing the weight of your body to press the ball into the trigger point. Hold for 8 to 12 seconds and continue to trigger point as usual.

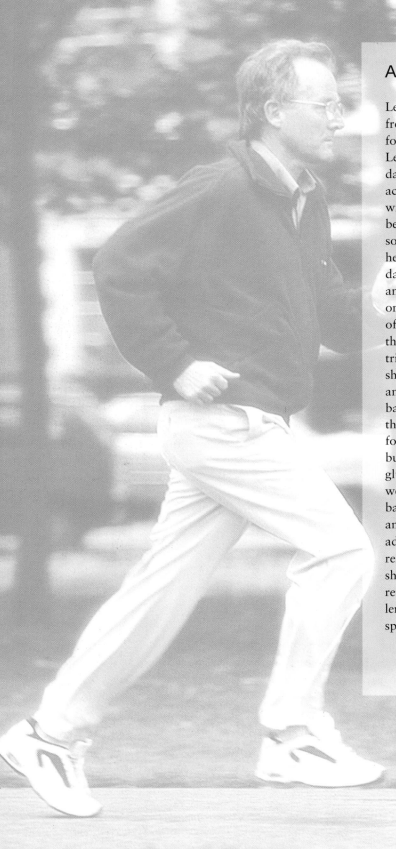

A story of low back pain

Les, an ex-firefighter, had been suffering from low back pain for many years following an accident at work. As far as Les was concerned, his lower back was damaged and nobody could help him. In actual fact, Les's pain had little to do with the muscles in his back, but was being referred to his back from another source. Due to the nature of the injury he had sustained at work, Les had damaged a deep muscle in his hip called an iliopsoas. This had a double impact on Les. Firstly, the subsequent shortening of the muscle had caused compression to the bones in his lower back. Secondly, trigger points had formed in the shortened and tense iliopsoas muscle, and these were firing pain signals into his back. Also, due to the lack of mobility that had ensued, trigger points had formed in the smaller muscles of the buttock region (the gluteus medius and gluteus minimus). These trigger points were also referring pain to his lower back area, as well as into the buttocks and the back of his leg, all of which added to his pain and discomfort. By removing the trigger points in the shortened stressed muscles and then returning them to their normal resting length, Les was freed from pain in the space of a few days.

Step 3: Elongate

Once the muscle has been irrigated and any trigger points in it have been eradicated, the muscle must next be returned to its normal length. While a muscle is tight, nerves can be trapped and pressure in the joints can increase, causing restriction and degeneration. The importance of stretching and maintaining your muscles' normal length cannot be overlooked. Even with adequate amounts of blood and the eradication of trigger points, if the muscle is not then lengthened the whole cycle of dysfunction can start again. The restriction in the muscle limits blood flow, and this allows waste products to build up. These toxins, along with the increase of muscular tension and decrease of muscle function, cause trigger points to be formed. The trigger points cause the muscle to tighten and you're right back where you started. Muscle tightness, as well as being a major cause of pain and discomfort is also a major contributor to postural distortion. This can be incredibly destructive to the stability and proper movement of your body.

There are many different ways to stretch. One of the simplest and easiest methods is the static stretch. This involves stretching your muscles until you feel only slight discomfort and holding this position for 15 to 20 seconds. After a short rest, this is repeated until you have stretched the muscle five times. When stretching, keep in mind that you are putting increased stress on the muscles; do not overstretch, and never make bouncing movements. Just hold the stretch steady.

Another type of stretching, which is explained and used in Part Four, is a form of isometric

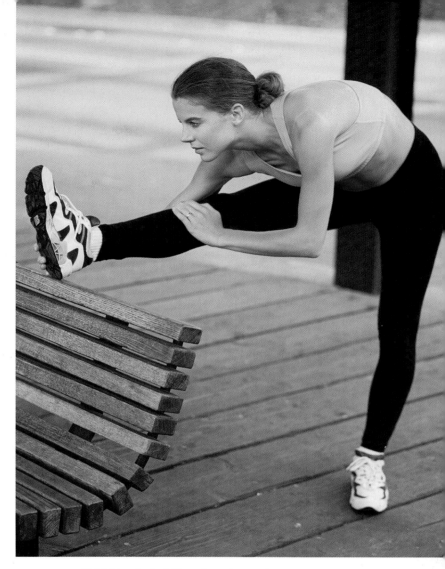

Maintaining the flexibility and suppleness of your muscles is one of the best ways in which to safeguard them against injury, pain, and dysfunction.

stretching. This type of stretching, sometimes known as muscle energy techniques (M.E.T.), involves contracting the muscles gently before the static stretch. Although it takes a bit of time to get used to M.E.T., it has been included as the method of choice for several reasons. As well as lengthening tight muscles, this method of stretching has been shown to help remove trigger points, normalize nerve impulses to and from muscles, and improve the tone of the treated muscles.

How often should you treat the area?

You can massage (irrigate) and stretch (elongate) every day if you wish. However, it is sensible to treat trigger points (eradicate) only every two to three days. The reason for this is that after trigger point treatment, the areas being treated can sometimes become quite sore and a little inflamed, particularly the first couple of times. This discomfort—if it does happen—should only last a day or so, after which the whole area will start to feel much better. Leaving a day or two in between each treatment allows this minor inflammation to settle before treatment begins again. There is no hard and fast rule for how many treatments are needed to eradicate any given trigger point, some will disperse after just one treatment while others may need to be treated nine or ten times. Just keep treating the affected muscles until the trigger points have gone and the muscles have returned to their normal, pain-free state. It should also be noted that although many trigger points can easily be treated by yourself it is often useful and, especially where the back is concerned, preferable to get someone to work the area for you. This can be a friend, a professional neuromuscular therapist, or you could even take this book along to a massage therapist and ask him or her to work on the necessary areas.

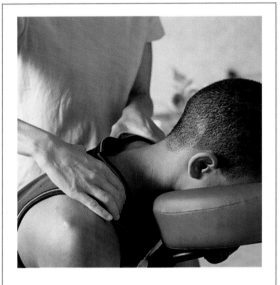

In certain parts of your body, such as your back and some parts of your shoulder, the muscles can be a little hard to get to on your own. If you can't reach the muscle yourself simply get someone else to work the muscle for you. Don't worry too much about accuracy; the pain will guide you to the correct spots. Alternatively, if you really are working by yourself, you can simply use the stretching and toning exercises in Part Four by themselves. This is approach is still extremely effective but may just take a little longer to achieve results.

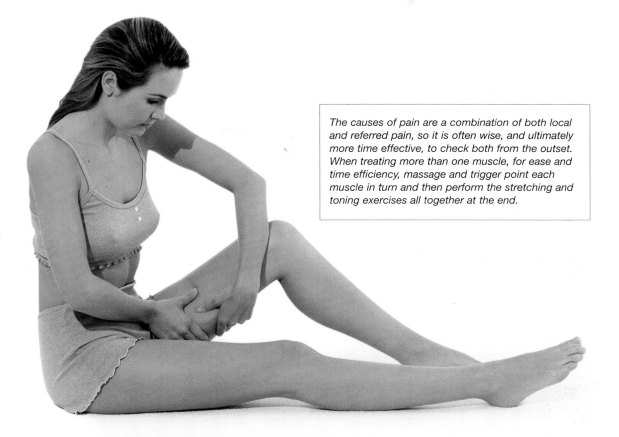

The causes of pain are a combination of both local and referred pain, so it is often wise, and ultimately more time effective, to check both from the outset. When treating more than one muscle, for ease and time efficiency, massage and trigger point each muscle in turn and then perform the stretching and toning exercises all together at the end.

A simple pain-relief strategy

The specifics of pain-relief treatment are best illustrated through example; in this case imagine that you had a pain in your upper thigh.

The simplest approach for relieving the pain is as follows. Using the anatomical diagrams for leg muscles as a guide (see Part Three), begin to gently treat the painful muscles using the three-step approach: irrigate – eradicate – elongate.

After the first two steps (massaging the painful area and removing trigger points) one of two things will happen.

Scenario A

There may be several areas in one or more of these muscles that are causing you pain. Continue to massage these affected areas, remove trigger points, and elongate the relevant muscles using the stretching and toning exercises in Part Four. The pain should ease within a few days.

Scenario B

You may find that these muscles, although tender, do not seem to be causing you specific pain, or that after three to four days of treatment, you are not getting any relief. This is a strong indication the pain is being referred from other muscles. If this is the case, go back to the pain referral pictures in Part Three. Match the shaded areas on the photographs with the areas in which you are feeling pain or discomfort. The diagrams will tell you which muscles could be causing your particular problems (in this case the Adductor longus, Deep rotators, Iliopsoas, and Rectus femoris). Massage each of these muscles in turn, and you will most likely find that at least one of them will feel painful. Don't forget to check the pain-referral zones of muscles in all parts of your body, as pain in the legs could be referred from your back or pelvis, for example. When you have identified all the muscles that seem to be causing you pain, continue with your cycle of irrigate – eradicate – elongate on all of them.

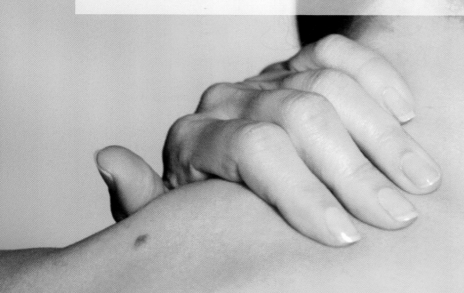

Summary points

- If a muscle is sore then it's an indication that it is probably restricted and receiving limited blood supply.

- Blocking pain through the use of analgesics or painkillers is useful in some circumstances, but does not get to the root of the problem and, therefore, is not a long-term solution.

- Relieving pain by eliminating its cause is, by far, the most effective solution to pain.

- Treat serious injuries in which you might have internal bleeding using the Rest – Ice – Compression – Elevation formula or by visiting your doctor.

- If there is no risk of bleeding around a painful muscle, joint, or tendon, begin to treat the cause by increasing blood supply to the area. Use massage or apply heat to achieve this.

- If a muscle "triggers" pain, discomfort, or other sensations to other parts of your body when pressed, then this is an indication that your nervous system is overloaded. Look for trigger points and eradicate them by applying pressure.

- Look for other muscles that could be referring pain into the area by using the pain-referral photographs in Part Three.

- Stretch the muscles and tone the opposing muscles using the appropriate exercises in Part Four.

- Remember that pain is only a symptom. It is a warning and as such you can learn a great deal from it.

Preventing pain from re-occurring

Although working on removing pain and discomfort is most definitely a worthwhile endeavor, it can sometimes be, in itself, a symptomatic approach. Even when you've eliminated the pain, there may still be an underlying cause that, if not addressed, can lead to the pain returning or even to new aches, pains, and injuries. Indeed, in some pain patterns, especially when the problem is many years old, even the above strategies for pain relief may not be enough to release you from pain until you have addressed all the underlying postural distortions.

In a perfect world, you would not be coming to BodySmart from a position of pain. The most effective approach would be to rebalance your body before pain and dysfunction occur and to use the tools contained in this book to strengthen and improve, not just to fix and patch. Structural body mapping, in the next chapter, will allow you to identify the areas where your body is holding the most tension. Then, using the same techniques you learned in this chapter to eradicate pain, you can begin to restore your body's natural balance. By recognizing potential imbalances, you can help safeguard against future problems.

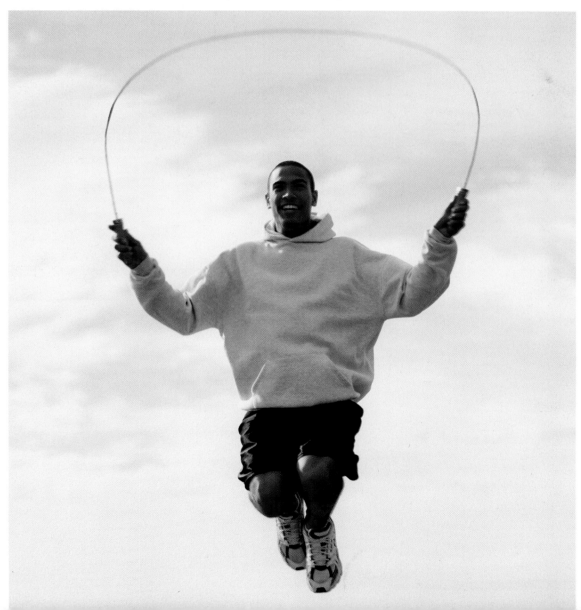

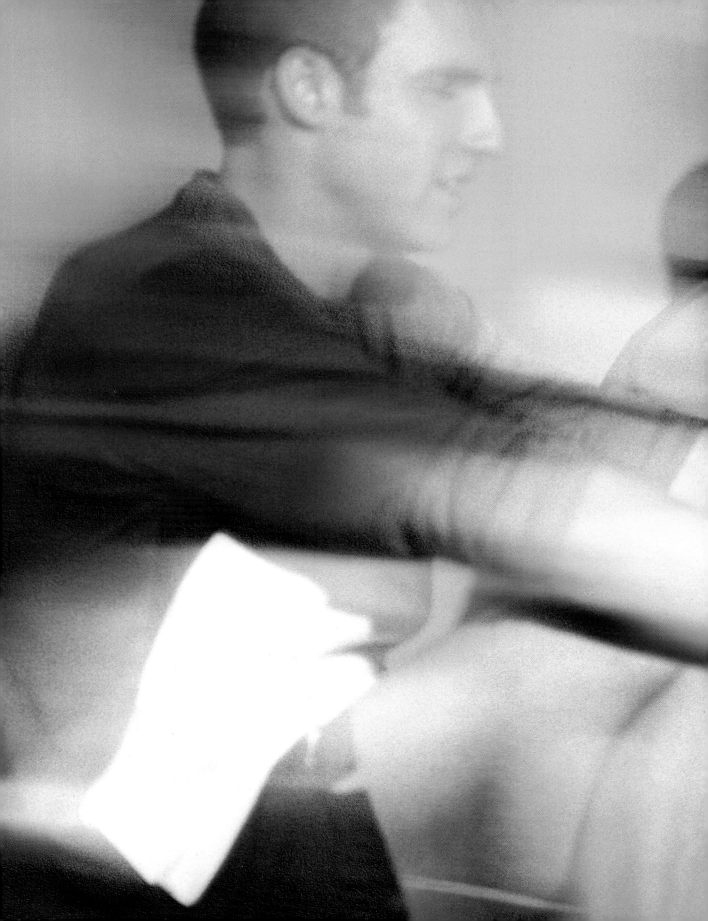

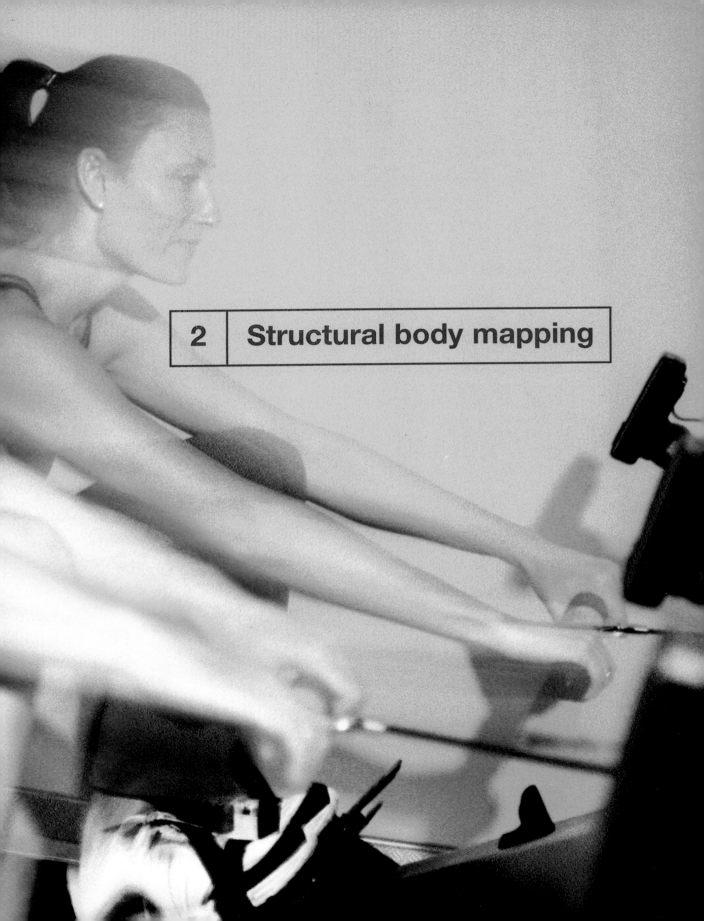

2 | **Structural body mapping**

Steps to body mapping

Whenever muscles become tight, the risk of movement restriction, pain, and discomfort increases. Constricted muscles and their faulty patterns often show up in your posture even before you're aware that a problem exists, so the key to a strong, healthy body is being able to spot these signs in advance and remedy them.

If muscles become tight and restricted, several undesirable things can start to happen, both in the immediate area and throughout the body:

- The nerves running through these muscles become compressed, which often leads to pain and discomfort.
- If left untreated, constricted muscles can start to form trigger points, which relay pain signals to other parts of the body (see pages 34–5).
- Shortened muscles can lead to postural distortions. These, in turn, cause a knock-on effect across the body and place additional strain on your joints, leading to limited movement and possibly further pain.
- If ignored, postural distortions can lead to joint deterioration.
- Incorrect posture and tightened muscles can increase the body's susceptibility to injury, particularly in athletes.

Reading your body

This chapter will show you a unique, step-by-step sequence, known as structural body mapping, which will enable you to "read" your

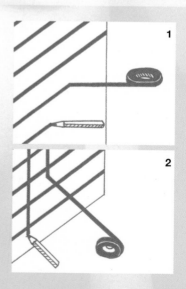

CREATING THE GRID

For the most accurate self-measurements, you will need the following items:

- black masking tape or a thick, black marker pen
- a full-length mirror
- a tape measure
- a spirit level

1 Using the masking tape or marker pen draw horizontal lines across the whole mirror at 4-inch (10-cm) intervals. Use the spirit level to ensure the lines are perfectly horizontal.

2 Then draw vertical lines down the length of the mirror. Mark them out at regular 4-inch (10-cm) intervals, to finish with a lattice-like pattern. Your grid is now complete.

3 Stand at least 6 to 8 feet (2 to 2.5 m) away from the mirror, so you can see your full-length reflection from head to toe.

4 Check that you're standing on a level surface. An uneven floor will deceive your eye and give you a misleading reading. If the floor dips in places, put down a wooden plank and, using the spirit level for accuracy, prop up one end to level off the surface.

own body—or that of a partner—and decipher its individual code. On the following pages you will learn how to assess the different areas of your body: your pelvis, shoulders, head and neck, legs, and spine. For a complete picture you need to map your body from the front, the side, and the back. The following process will allow you to make an accurate assessment of your posture.

Begin by drawing up a mirrored grid (see box, page 50). This will help you decide exactly how and where there are any distortions in your body. If you're working with a partner, a plumb line (see box, below) will be sufficient.

For best results avoid loose, flowing clothes. Strip down to your underwear in order to see what you are trying to measure, without the distraction of extra layers of clothing.

Stand in a normal, relaxed position. Check the position of your feet and make sure that one foot is not farther forward than the other. If you are working on your own, stand with your navel in line with one of the vertical lines on your grid.

When working with a partner, the plumb line will serve as your central line.

Take each measurement in turn, as described on pages 52–60. Mark your results, then remember to return to a natural stance before the next stage. For measurements that are difficult to take on your own, such as mapping your head and neck from the side, ask a friend to help or use a camera with a self-timer. If you are working with a partner, make sure the person taking the measurements keeps his/her head straight, eyes level with hands, when measuring the horizontal plane of your shoulders or pelvic alignment.

If you notice a distortion, put a check in the corresponding box on the posture chart on pages 52–3. Indicate on which side of your body the misalignment occurs: L for left; R for right. If there is a misalignment on both sides, check both boxes. In some areas you may have more than one type of distortion; in others you may have none, and so check none of the boxes.

When body mapping, check your whole body for postural deviations, don't just concentrate on the part or parts that feel painful. This is because the body has a natural tendency toward the knock-on effect (see pages 25–7) and even if you treat those parts of your body where you feel discomfort, there may be other underlying causes at work. If you ignore the causes, your symptoms may later return or show up as distortions in other parts of your body.

MAKING YOUR PLUMB LINE

You will need the following items to make a plumb line:
- a long piece of string
- a small, weighted object such as a box of matches
- a thumbtack

1 Securely tie one end of the string around a box of matches or other weighted object.

2 Using the tack, attach the other end of the string to the ceiling. Make sure that the weight you are using hangs clear of the floor by about 1 inch (2.5 cm). Use it to gauge an exact vertical line.

3 Position your feet behind the plumb line so they are level.

Using your body map

Once you have assessed your whole body, you can start finding out more about the causes of any problems and how to treat them.

- Once you have filled in the chart, right, turn to pages 61–5 for more information on the postural distortions. The check boxes relate directly to the distortions outlined in this section. For example, if you check Shoulder A in the chart, you should turn to Shoulder A in the postural distortions section. These pages describe the distortion in detail, tell you which muscles are causing it, and whether any other muscles may be affected.

- You should first treat any pain and then use the recommended stretches to address the underlying problem. If you have pain, in the area of shoulder, for example, massage the muscles indicated for this area using the Irrigate – Eradicate – Elongate techniques outlined on pages 38–44.

- If you are having trouble locating the pain, or it is not easing, it may be a result of referred pain. Turn to Part Three, the Pain Referral section, and match the shaded zones with the area/s of your body where you are feeling discomfort. Identify the causative muscles using the corresponding anatomical illustrations. Finally, turn to the relevant stretching and toning exercises in Part Four to elongate the tightened muscle/s.

- Even if you don't have any pain, keep in mind that distortions can affect everyday movements or your performance in certain sports. There is more information on exactly which sports and movements are affected in the athletic performance charts following the descriptions of the distortions. The stretching and toning exercises in Part Four will help you remedy any problems.

PELVIS

	L	R
A	☐	☐
B	☐	☐
C	☐	☐
D	☐	☐
E	☐	☐
F		
G		

Note: When you are putting checks inside the chart boxes, indicate the side of the body on which the misalignment occurred (L for left; R for right). If there was a misalignment on both sides, check both boxes.

SHOULDERS		HEAD AND NECK		LEGS		SPINE	
L ☐	R ☐	L ☑	R ☑	L ☐	R ☐	L ☐	R ☐
L ☐	R ☐	L ☑	R ☑	L ☐	R ☐	L ☐	R ☐
L ☐	R ☐	L ☑	R ☑			L ☐	R ☐
L ☐	R ☐					L ☐	R ☐
L ☐	R ☐					L ☐	R ☐
L ☐	R ☐					L ☐	R ☐
L ☐	R ☐						

ARCHES

L ☐	R ☐

If you checked an Arches box, you have determined that the arches of one or both of your feet may have dropped. A dropped arch can have a big effect on your posture, so you should visit a chiropodist or podiatrist to be measured for arch supports for your shoes. Dropped arches can help to perpetuate forward rotation of the pelvis and "set" many postural distortions in place.

Mapping from the front

Stand in a relaxed position in front of the mirrored grid with your feet level and shoulder-width apart.

Mapping your pelvis

To check the horizontal level of your hips, gently push your hands into your waist so that they rest on top of the pelvic bone. If you're working with a partner, crouch in front of him/her so that your eyes are level with your fingers when you take this measurement.

If one side of the pelvis seems higher than the other, put a check in the box marked Pelvis A for that side.

Next, gently push your thumbs into the front of your hips and circle them until you have located the two small bones at the front of your pelvis. Look down to check whether one thumb is further forward than the other.

If one of the thumbs is further forward, put a check in the box marked Pelvis D for that side.

Mapping your shoulders

Look at the horizontal grid lines on the mirror to assess the plane of your shoulders. If you're working with a partner, use the bony notch on each of his/her shoulders as measuring points. If one of these points is higher than the other, you may have either a raised or depressed shoulder, both of which indicate muscle imbalance. Also, examine the line of the collarbones (which should be fairly level). If they seem to be angled up on the side of the higher shoulder, this shows a raised shoulder. If one collarbone appears to be angled down on the side that dips, this shows a depressed shoulder.

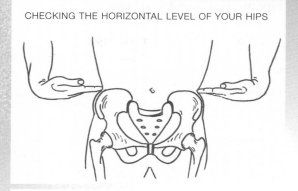

CHECKING THE HORIZONTAL LEVEL OF YOUR HIPS

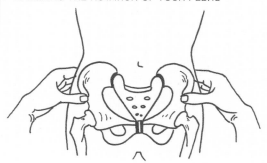

CHECKING THE ROTATION OF YOUR PELVIS

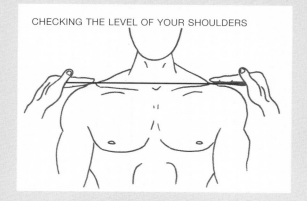

CHECKING THE LEVEL OF YOUR SHOULDERS

Mapping your head and neck

Use the vertical line that runs through the center of your reflection to determine whether your head is straight or cocked to one side. If you're working with a partner, check that the plumb line hangs in front of your partner's navel and look to see whether or not his/her head is straight or tilted.

If the head is tilted to one side, put a check in the box marked Head and Neck A for that side.

Use the plumb line or the central line of the mirrored grid to determine whether or not the head is turned to one side.

If the head is rotated to one side, put a check in the box marked Head and Neck C for that side.

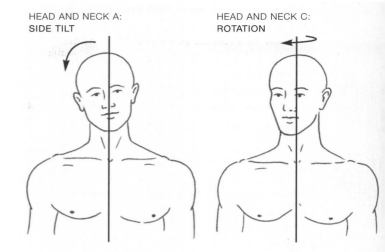

HEAD AND NECK A:
SIDE TILT

HEAD AND NECK C:
ROTATION

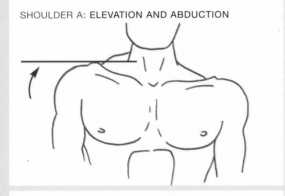

SHOULDER A: ELEVATION AND ABDUCTION

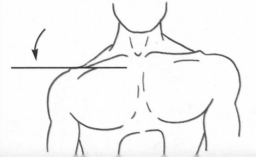

SHOULDER B: DEPRESSION AND ADDUCTION

If one shoulder is higher than the other, put a check in the box marked Shoulder A for the raised side.

If one shoulder is lower than the other, put a check in the box marked Shoulder B for the lowered side.

Now let your hands hang naturally down by your sides.

If the backs of your hands are turning toward the front, put a check in the box marked Shoulder C.

If the palms of your hands are turning toward the front, put a check in the box marked Shoulder D.

Mapping from the side

Turn to the side, aligning the right side of your body to the grid or plumb line using your ankle bone as a reference point (see picture, right). It is more reliable than using your shoulders or your ear, as any distortions you have may push these into the wrong positions.

Mapping your pelvis

Again, as it is the source of many other distortions in the body, begin with your pelvis. First, check for forward or backward rotation of the pelvis. Press the front of your pelvis until you find small protruding bones. Then look for the prominent bone (the posterior iliac spine, see picture, far right) that juts out slightly from your back, about 1–2 inches (2–2.5 cm) on either side of the base of your spine. Gently circle your fingers until you locate this bone.

Position your fingers just underneath these bones with your fingers straight and the tips pointing toward each other. Imagine your fingers are extended and can actually touch in the middle. The angle they are at will tell you if there is any rotation in the pelvis. The normal position is 5–10 forward degrees for women and 0–5 forward degrees for men. If your fingers are farther forward than these positions then the pelvis is fowardly rotated; if they are farther back, the pelvis is backwardly rotated. If you're working alone, use the horizontal lines on the grid to help you assess whether there is pelvic rotation. If you're working on another person, keep your eyes at the same level as your fingers and avoid tilting your head when placing your fingers on either side of your partner's pelvis.

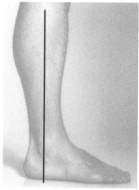
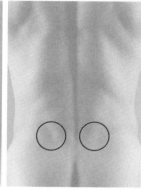

Stand so that the central vertical line aligns with the small bone on the side of your ankle.

The posterior iliac spine is marked by two indentations near the base of your spine (circled).

CHECKING FOR ROTATION OF YOUR PELVIS

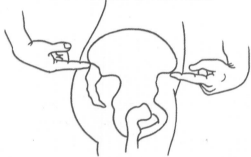

CHECKING YOUR PARTNER'S PELVIS

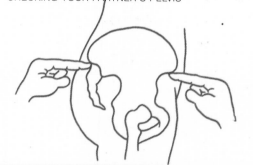

PELVIS B: FORWARD ROTATION

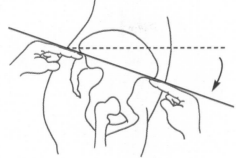

GOOD POSTURE WITH NO
PROJECTION OF THE PELVIS

PELVIS E: PROJECTION

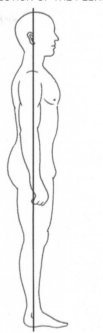

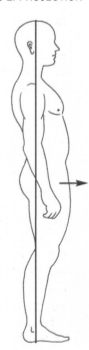

PELVIS C: BACKWARD ROTATION

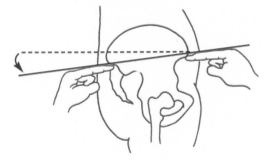

If the fingers tilt forward (more than 10 degrees for a woman and more than 5 degrees for a man), put a check in the box marked Pelvis B.

If the fingers are positioned at less than 5 degrees (for a woman) or tilted backward from the horizontal (for a man), put a check in the box marked Pelvis C.

Now check that your ankle still aligns with the central line of the grid or the plumb line. Look at your hips to see if they are being pushed forward of this line or not.

If your hips are being thrust forward, put a check in the box marked Pelvis E.

Now turn around and repeat all the measurements on your left side.

If your pelvis was rotated forward, it is likely that the arches of your feet have started to drop. Put a check in the box marked Arches.

Look at your knees. Are they locked back? A normal standing position requires that your knees be slightly bent. This will give you an idea whether you knees are at risk. As you rectify any distortions to your pelvis, your knees should move back into a normal position. The exercises shown on pages 106–7 and 147–8, to rectify a forward rotation of the hips, will also help stretch tightness around the knees.

Mapping your shoulders

Look closely at the shape of your shoulder blade.

If your shoulder blade sticks out or looks winged (with the bottom edge of your shoulder blade lifted away from your back), put a check in the box marked Shoulder G.

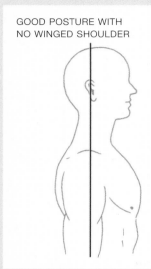

GOOD POSTURE WITH NO WINGED SHOULDER

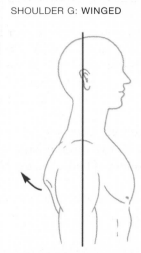

SHOULDER G: WINGED

Mapping your head and neck

Examine whether or not your head is correctly positioned by checking to see if your ear lines up with your shoulder through the plumb line. This is one of the few measurements that is difficult to take for yourself; you could use a camera with a self-timer to take a photograph of your head and neck from the side. Use this to check whether you have a forward head position.

If your ear comes further forward than your shoulder, put a check in the box marked Head and Neck B for the appropriate side.

However, there is another way to tell if you have a forward head position. If your hips are rotated forward (see page 57), there is a very strong likelihood that your head is in a forward position, too, due to the knock-on effect.

If there is a forward rotation of the pelvis, put a check in the box marked Head and Neck B.

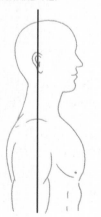

GOOD POSTURE WITH NO PROTRUSION AND BACKWARD TILT

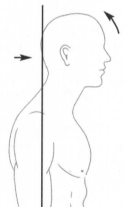

HEAD AND NECK B: PROTRUSION AND BACKWARD TILT

Mapping from the back

Since you need to see your back for these measurements, you need to use a camera with a self-timer if you cannot find a partner to help you. However, the front of your body also gives you hints about what's happening at the back.

Mapping your shoulders

Look at your upper back area and check the position of both shoulder blades.

If your shoulder blades are drawn in toward your spine, put a check in the box marked Shoulder E.

If your shoulder blades are pulled away from your spine, put a check in the box marked Shoulder F.

Note: If your shoulder blade is being drawn in toward your spine, then when seen from the front it will often appear that your shoulder is being drawn backward and your chest pushed forward. If your shoulder blade is being pulled away from your spine, from the front it will often appear that your shoulder has become hunched forward and your chest is sunken.

SHOULDER E: RETRACTION

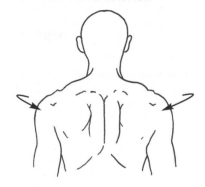

SHOULDER F: PROTRACTION

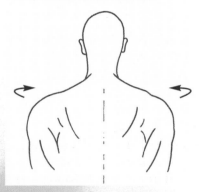

Mapping your legs

Looking at the bottom of your calf muscle, you will see a tendon protruding for about 2 inches (5 cm) up from the top of your heel. This is your Achilles tendon. If it is noticeably curving in toward the inside of your leg, this indicates that the arches of your feet may have dropped.

If your Achilles tendon is curving in toward the inside of your leg, put a check in the box marked Arches.

Finally, assess your walking pattern. Walk in a straight line and note the positions of your feet.

If one or both of your feet are turned outward when walking, put a check in the box marked Leg A.

If one or both of your feet are turned inward when walking, put a check in the box marked Leg B.

Mapping your spine

After mapping your pelvis, shoulders, head, and legs, you can assess what is happening with your spine. This is because the posture of your back relates directly to the position of your pelvis and shoulders. Using the information from the rest of the posture chart, work through the checklist on the right to fill in the spine section accordingly.

To treat the spine successfully, always rectify the distortions in the shoulders and hips first. Once these underlying causes have been rectified, stretch the affected spinal muscles for several weeks to further release the back.

Identifying postural distortions

After mapping your body and filling in the posture charts, you will be able to identify the distortions that are occurring. The following pages contain information on each distortion pattern of the pelvis, shoulders, neck, spine, and legs.

For each pattern there is a brief description of the distortion and a list of the primary muscles pulling the bones out of alignment. The muscles listed as "also affected" are not directly involved in the distortion but can shorten as a result of it, leading to possible dysfunction and the formation of trigger points. You will also find details of movements that may be affected by the distortions, and examples of sports in which performance may be impaired by them.

Were your shoulders level but not your hips?
Put a check in the box marked Spine A on the side corresponding to the higher hip.

Were your shoulders and hips raised on the same side (e.g. your right shoulder and right hip)?
Put a check in the box marked Spine B on the side on which your shoulder and hip were raised.

Were your shoulders and hips raised on different sides (e.g. your left shoulder and right hip)?
Put a check in the box marked Spine C on the side on which your hip was raised.

Were your shoulders uneven but your hips level?
Put a check in the box marked Spine A on the side on which your shoulder was held higher, regardless of whether you found it to be anatomically raised (Shoulder A) or lowered (Shoulder B).

Were your hips rotated forward (Pelvis B)?
Put a check in the box marked Spine E for the corresponding side.

Were your hips rotated backward (Pelvis C)?
Put a check in the box marked Spine F for the corresponding side.

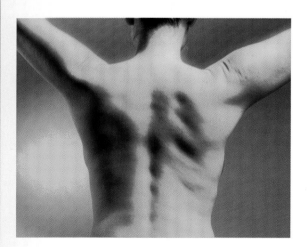

Postural distortions of the pelvis

	MUSCLES THAT CAN BECOME RESTRICTED	ASSOCIATED MOVEMENTS	SPORTS AFFECTED
Pelvis A (side tilt) One hip is higher than the other, pulling the leg bone (femur) on the raised side slightly toward the center	Quadratus lumborum, External oblique, Internal oblique Also affected: Adductor longus, Adductor brevis, Adductor magnus, Pectineus, Iliopsoas	These muscles are used during side bending, twisting, and throwing, and when raising your legs or doing sit-ups. They also stabilize the spine when you lift heavy weights	**Baseball** (pitching, hitting); **Tennis** (serving, smash shots); **Volleyball** (the spike); **Martial arts Javelin; Gymnastics; Golf; Bodybuilding; Powerlifting; Cricket** (bowling, hitting)
Pelvis B (forward rotation) The front of your pelvis is pulled down and the back is lifted up, causing the pelvis to rotate forward	Adductor longus, Gracilis, Pectineus, Rectus femoris Also affected: Erector spinae, Quadratus lumborum, Tensor fasciae	These muscles are used in side-stepping, side-lunging, bringing your leg toward your body from the side, raising your knees and extending your legs, and kicking a ball with the instep	**Football** and **Rugby** (side-stepping); **Soccer** (passing); **Jumping; Running; Hurdles; Martial arts; Tennis; Basketball; Volleyball; Swimming** (breaststroke)
Pelvis C (backward rotation) The front of your pelvis is lifted up and the back is pulled down, causing the pelvis to rotate backward	Biceps femoris, Semitendinosus, Semimembranosus (the hamstring group), Rectus abdominus Also affected: Gluteus maximus, External obliques, Iliopsoas	The first three of these muscles are used in bending the knee when running, jumping, lunging and pulling the thigh backward. The Rectus abdominus is used in sit-ups, when throwing, and when lifting your legs to the front	**Football** (throwing, running, kicking); **Soccer** (lunge tackle); **Baseball** (pitching); **Tennis** (lunging); **Cricket** (throwing); **Gymnastics; Martial arts; Running; Swimming** (kicking); **Weight lifting**
Pelvis D (horizontal twist) One side of your pelvis is pushed farther forward than the other.	External and Internal obliques Also affected: Iliopsoas, Rotatores, Multifidi	These muscles are used during side bending, twisting, and throwing, and when raising your legs or doing sit-ups. They also stabilize the spine when you lift heavy weights	**Baseball** (throwing, hitting); **Tennis** (serving, smash shots); **Volleyball** (the spike); **Cricket** (bowling); **Martial arts; Golf; Gymnastics; Javelin; Bodybuilding; Powerlifting**
Pelvis E (projection) The whole of your pelvis is drawn forward, and you seem to "lead the way" with your hips	Biceps femoris, Erector spinae, Semitendinosus, Semimembranosus, Gluteus maximus, Quadratus lumborum Also affected:Multifidi, Rotatores	These muscles are used in bending the knee, pulling your thigh backward, and side bending, and they help stabilize the spine when you lift heavy weights or throw objects	**Running; Football; Soccer** (lunge tackle); **Tennis** (lunging); **Baseball** (pitching); **Gymnastics; Martial arts; Swimming; Cricket; Golf; Rowing; Weight lifting**

Postural distortions of the shoulder, head, and neck

	MUSCLES THAT CAN BECOME RESTRICTED	ASSOCIATED MOVEMENTS	SPORTS AFFECTED
Shoulder A (elevation) When your shoulder is held in this position, its outer edge is lifted up and slightly in toward your body (elevation). There can often be a secondary pattern in which its bottom angle is rotated away from your spine (abduction)	Upper trapezius, Levator scapulae, Serratus anterior (lower part) Also affected: Latissimus dorsi, Teres major, Teres minor	These muscles are all used when reaching upward overhead, e.g. stretching up high to catch, push, or hit an object. Trapezius and Levator scapulae: important for stabilizing the head, e.g. in gymnastics and boxing	**Football; Soccer** (goalkeeping); **Baseball** and **Cricket** (fielding); **Rugby** (line-outs); **Tennis** (serving, smash shots); **Volleyball** (the spike); **Basketball** (dunk); **Bodybuilding** (shoulder presses, shrugs); **Weight lifting** (cleans)
Shoulder B (depression) When your shoulder is in this position, its outer edge is moved down and slightly inward (depression). Often its bottom edge is rotated up and toward your spine (adduction)	Latissimus dorsi, Lower trapeziius, Pectoralis minor (if shoulder is winged), Erector spinae Also affected: Supraspinatus	These muscles are used in throwing, and when pulling yourself upward. Latissimus dorsi: used when pulling your arms back horizontally from the front. Pectoralis minor: used when pushing down against resistance. Erector spinae: primarily supports and stabilizes spine	**Gymnastics** (horizontal bar, rings); **Swimming; Rowing; Judo; Tennis; Climbing; Basketball** (dunk); **Baseball** (pitching); **Cricket** (bowling); **Volleyball** (the spike); **Bodybuilding** (lat pull-downs, chins)
Shoulder C (internal rotation) When your shoulder is in this position, your arm rotates in toward your body (internal rotation)	Pectoralis major, Subscapularis, Teres major Also affected: Latissimus dorsi	Tightness leads to problems turning arm inward, drawing arm over head and behind to throw, and drawing arm across body, e.g. in hugging or pushing	**Football** and **Rugby** (tackling, pushing); **Tennis** (forehand); **Baseball** (pitching); **Cricket; Rowing; Boxing; Martial arts; Swimming;**
Shoulder D (external rotation) In this position, your arm rotates away from your body (external rotation)	Infraspinatus, Teres minor	External rotation is needed when an arm is drawn backward to throw. Tightness can cause obstruction to opposing muscles that turn arm inward.	**Tennis** (backhand); **Baseball** (pitching); **Cricket** (fielding); **Boxing, Martial arts** (various strikes); **Swimming; Weight lifting; Gymnastics**
Shoulder E (retraction) In this position, your shoulder blade is pulled across your back toward your spine (retraction)	Middle trapezius, Lower trapezius, Latissimus dorsi (upper part), Rhomboids	All involved in bringing shoulder blades together, e.g. when pulling arms back horizontally from the front, as in many throwing actions. Middle and Lower trapezius: help you to reach upward	**Baseball** (pitching); **Cricket** (fielding); **Rowing; Tennis** (backhand); **Archery; Judo** (pulling); **Boxing, Martial arts** (drawing the arm to strike); **Swimming** (breaststroke)

	MUSCLES THAT CAN BECOME RESTRICTED	ASSOCIATED MOVEMENTS	SPORTS AFFECTED
Shoulder F (protraction) When your shoulder is held in this position, your shoulder blade is moved across your back, away from your spine (protraction)	Serratus anterior, Pectoralis minor Also affected: Pectoralis major	Both used when pushing an object forward, which requires shoulder blades to protract (flare out). Serratus anterior: used when reaching upward. Pectoralis minor: stabilizes shoulder blade when pushing down against resistance	**Football** (pushing, blocking); **Weight lifting** (bench-pressing); **Gymnastics** (floorwork, parallel bars, rings); **Sumo wrestling** (warding off); **Boxing, Martial arts** (various front strikes)
Shoulder G (winged) The bottom edge of your shoulder blade is lifted away from your back, and the top part is often pulled slightly inward	Pectoralis minor	Used when bringing arms from over head to your sides or pulling your body upward; stabilizes shoulder blade when pushing down against resistance	**Football** (pushing, blocking); **Weight lifting** (bench-pressing); **Gymnastics** (floorwork, rings, bars); **Boxing; Martial arts; Swimming** (front crawl); **Climbing**
Head and neck A (side tilt/lateral flexion) When your neck is held in this position, your head is pulled over to one side	Upper trapezius, Sternocleidomastoid, Semispinalis cervicus, Multifidi, Scalenes Also affected: Semispinalis capitis, Levator scapulae	Upper trapezius:reaching over head to catch, push, or hit an object. Sternocleidomastoid: helps brace neck against impact. Scalenes: vital for correct and deep breathing	**Football; Rugby; Soccer** (heading); **Basketball** (dunk); **Tennis** (serving, smash shots); **Volleyball** (spike); **Boxing,** and **Martial arts** (impact resistance); **Swimming; Cricket** (fielding)
Head and neck B (protrusion) When your neck is held in this position, your head is pushed forward and tilts back slightly	Sternocleidomastoid, Scalenes (anterior head) Also affected: Semispinalis capitis, Rectus capitis posterior major, Splenius capitis, Splenius cervicis, Longus capitis, Longus colli	Sternocleidomastoid: helps brace neck against impact, for example when heading a soccer ball. Scalenes: vital for correct and deep breathing	**Soccer** (heading the ball); **Football, Rugby, Boxing, Martial arts** (impact resistance); **Swimming; Tennis** (spatial awareness)
Head and neck C (rotation) When your neck is held in this position, your head is turned to one side	Sternocleidomastoid, Splenius capitis, Splenius cervicis, Rectus capitis posterior major, Obliquus capitis inferior	Sternocleidomastoid: helps brace neck against impact, for example when heading a soccer ball	**Soccer** (heading the ball); **Football, Rugby, Boxing, Martial arts** (impact resistance); **Swimming** (turning the head to breathe in front crawl); **Tennis** (following the ball)

Postural distortions of the spine and legs

	MUSCLES THAT CAN BECOME RESTRICTED	ASSOCIATED MOVEMENTS	SPORTS AFFECTED
Spine A (shoulders level, hips tilted) The lower part of your spine bends to one side and straightens nearer the shoulders	Pelvic (hip) tilt: see **Pelvis A**, page 61 Affected spinal muscles: Erector spinae, Multifidi, Rotatores	Erector spinae: supports and stabilizes the spine. Used in extending spine backward. Multifidi, Rotatores: important for pain-free, unrestricted rotation of the spine	**Rowing**; **Baseball** (hitting); **Tennis** (twisting); **Martial arts** (various strikes, blocks, kicks); **Golf** (swing); **Weight lifting**; **Gymnastics**
Spine B (shoulders tilted, hips tilted on same side) When your shoulders and hips are held in this position, both are raised on the same side	Spine B and C Shoulders tilted: see **Shoulder A**, page 62 (elevation); **Shoulder B**, page 62 (depression) Pelvic hip tilt: see **Pelvis A**, page 61 Affected spinal muscles: Erector spinae, Multifidi, Rotatores	Spine B, C, and D Erector spinae: Supports and stabilizes the spine. Important when under major stress (e.g. in squatting and dead-lifting). Used in extending spine backward. Multifidi, Rotatores: important for pain-free, unrestricted rotation of the spine	**Rowing**; **Baseball** (hitting); **Tennis** (twisting); **Martial arts** (various strikes, blocks, kicks); **Golf** (swing); **Weight lifting**; **Gymnastics**
Spine C (shoulders tilted, hips tilted on opposite side) When your shoulders and hips are held in this position, they are raised on opposite sides			**Rowing**; **Baseball** (hitting); **Tennis** (twisting); **Martial arts** (various strikes, blocks, kicks); **Golf** (swing); **Weight lifting**; **Gymnastics**
Spine D (shoulders tilted, hips level) The lower part of your spine remains straight while the upper part bends to one side	Shoulder tilted: see **Shoulder A**, page 62 (elevation); **Shoulder B**, page 62 (depression) Affected spinal muscles: Erector spinae, Multifidi, Rotatores		**Rowing**; **Baseball** (hitting); **Tennis** (twisting); **Martial arts** (various strikes, blocks, kicks); **Golf** (swing); **Weight lifting**; **Gymnastics**
Spine E (lumbar curve) The lower part of your spine becomes overly curved (lordosis) and the spinal muscles on both sides become tight	Lumbar curve: see **Pelvis B**, page 61 Affected spinal muscles: Erector spinae, Multifidi, Rotatores Also affected: Iliopsoas	Erector spinae: supports, stabilizes, and extends spine backward. Multifidi, Rotatores: Important for pain-free, unrestricted rotation of the spine. Iliopsoas: running, kicking, lifting leg to front	**Rowing**; **Baseball** (hitting); **Tennis**; **Martial arts**; **Golf**; **Soccer**; **Rugby**; **Basketball**; **Volleyball** (jumping); **Running**; **Jumping**; **Diving** (tuck); **Weight lifting**; **Gymnastics**
Spine F (thoracic curve) Upper part of spine is overly curved (kyphosis) and the front of your body collapses slightly	Thoracic curve: see **Pelvis C**, page 61 Also affected: Rectus abdominis, External and internal obliques	All used when throwing, raising your legs to the front, and doing sit-ups. External and Internal obliques: used in side bending, throwing, lifting, and twisting	**Running**; **Football**; **Baseball** (pitching); **Gymnastics**; **Diving** (tuck); **Golf** (swing); **Tennis**; **Martial arts**; **Weight lifting**; **Cricket** (throwing)

	MUSCLES THAT CAN BECOME RESTRICTED	ASSOCIATED MOVEMENTS	SPORTS AFFECTED
Legs A (external rotation) In this position, the bone of your upper leg turns outward, away from your body, and the foot on that side points outward	Deep rotators (Superior and Inferior gemellus, Obturator internus and externus, Quadratus femoris), Piriformis, Gluteus maximus Also affected: Adductor longus, Adductor brevis, Adductor magnus (stretched together)	All externally rotate leg. Tightness can affect activities that involve turning the leg and foot outward. Gluteus maximus: for pulling leg back and for standing upright from bent-over position with locked knees	**Running** (sprinting, distance); **Soccer** (passing); **Gymnastics** (floor routines); **Martial arts** (various kicks); **Swimming** (kicking); **Weight lifting** (squats, dead-lifts); **Hurdles**; **Ice-skating**
Legs B (internal rotation) In this position, the bone of your upper leg turns in toward your body, and the foot on that side points inward	Gluteus medius, Gluteus minimus, Tensor fasciae latae, Semitendinosus, Semimembranosus Also affected: Iliopsoas	All internally rotate leg. Tightness can cause problems with turning the leg inward, lifting the leg to the side, side-stepping motions, and bending the knee	**Football, Rugby** (side-stepping, running); **Soccer** (dribbling); **Martial arts** (kicks); **Tennis** (side-lunging); **Running**; **Gymnastics; Swimming; Skiing**

Treating postural distortions

Good posture is vital for maintaining muscle balance and improving body shape. As well as reducing muscle tension, spasm, and pain, it reduces the risk of musculo-skeletal injuries and protects ligaments, tendons, and joints from undue mechanical stress.

It is quite common to have several postural distortions at any one time, and it can be confusing as to where to start first. It is best to address any distortions of the pelvis early on. It is often amazing how other distortions can rectify themselves if you reestablish balance in the pelvis.

The general order in which to treat structural distortions is as follows:

- First rectify the cause of any twisting or torque patterns (especially relevant if you checked Pelvis D on the posture chart).
- Next rectify any imbalances that interfere with the horizontal plane of your body, i.e. a raised/lowered shoulder or hip.
- Then deal with any muscular tightness that is pulling your body either forward or backward.

Once these have been dealt with, you can continue to put any other distortions right in whatever order you see fit. Treat all the muscles connected to a specific distortion pattern together in one collective exercise routine.

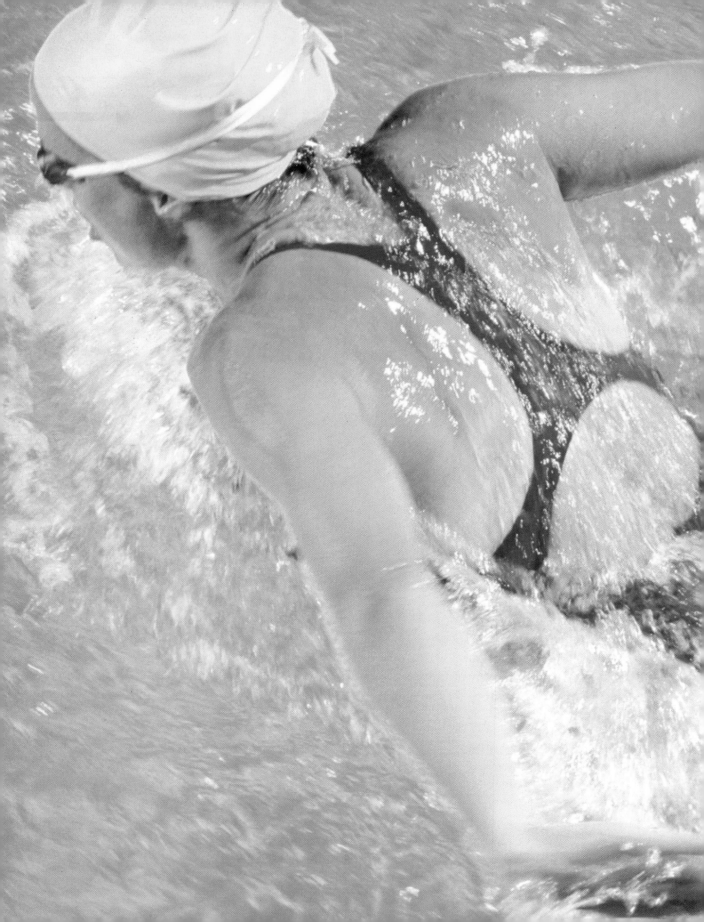

3 | Tight muscles and pain referral

Understanding muscles and pain

If you have mapped your body and identified distortions and tight muscles or if you are simply suffering pain in a particular area, it's useful to understand the characteristics of muscles before you start to treat them. This section will give you information on individual muscles and the areas to which they may refer pain.

This section is divided into the five key areas of the body: pelvis, shoulders, head and neck, legs, and back. Within each area you'll find muscle charts, detailing where individual muscles are located, the anatomy of the muscle, and how they are attached to the bones. Each entry is accompanied by information on what might have caused that muscle to become tight and restricted in the first place and the types of lifestyle activities you should avoid to prevent further tightness and injury. The shaded photographs show where you may be feeling pain as a result of injury or tightness in that muscle.

Using the charts

There are different ways to use the information in this section, depending on how you have used the rest of the book and whether you are suffering pain or not.

To treat distortions

If you have used Part Two to map your body, discovered distortions, and identified the muscles that are causing them, simply look up the relevant muscle entries by name to find out more about them.

Using the anatomical illustrations as a guide, you can then start to treat the muscles. Begin by gently massaging the area using the Irrigate – Eradicate – Elongate principle (see page 38). The exercises that will stretch the affected muscles and tone the opposing muscles are found in Part Four.

To treat pain

If you feel pain or discomfort in a particular muscle, it is important to treat the pain first. Once the pain has gone, or at least been greatly reduced, you will find it far easier to address the underlying postural problems.

As with treating a distortion, begin with the method Irrigate – Eradicate – Elongate (see page 38), using the information in this chapter to guide you, massaging each of the affected muscles in turn, and removing possible trigger points using the tenderness to guide you to the correct spot.

If you can't massage a particular muscle because it is out of your reach, and you have no one else who can help you, you can treat it with just the stretching and toning exercises, although sometimes this may take a little longer to relieve the pain. To further increase the effectiveness of the treatments, you can soak in a hot bath or take a warm shower before stretching.

By using the shaded areas on the photographs as a guide, you can locate which muscles may be causing your pain. Keep in mind that postural distortions can sometimes mask other pain patterns; although a particular muscle may feel tender to the touch, it may not be the cause of your discomfort. Therefore, you need to check all the muscles that refer pain to that site, as, even though you may have found one cause, there may be a combination of several injured muscles at play. For example, if you feel pain on the outside of your shoulder (in the Deltoid), you should consult the entries for the Infraspinatus, Latissimus dorsi, Levator scapulae, and the Pectoralis major, as pain can be referred into your shoulder from all of these muscles.

At the end of this chapter you will also find an easy reference chart of muscles that, although not directly connected to the area of pain, can still refer pain into that area.

Preventing further problems

You may be wondering what caused your muscle to become tight in the first place. Injury is one reason. Postural distortions are another: if one muscle pulls a bone out of alignment, this can lead to tightness in secondary muscles (these are listed in the postural distortions section, pages 61–5). However, seemingly innocuous everyday activities can also lead to stress and tightness. Once you have restored the natural balance to affected parts of your body, make good use of the What to Avoid lists under each entry to prevent you from re-injuring the muscle. It can be worthwhile glancing through all these lists to check that you are not putting other areas of the body at risk.

Understanding muscle descriptions

Each entry on the following pages includes a description of the anatomy and physiology of the muscle—in short, where it is and what it does. Remember that when a muscle contracts, one end keeps a fixed position while the other end moves. The end of your muscle that stays still is called the origin, and this can be thought of as the anchor point for the muscle. The other end, called the insertion, is the end of your muscle that moves and subsequently changes the position of the bone to which it is connected.

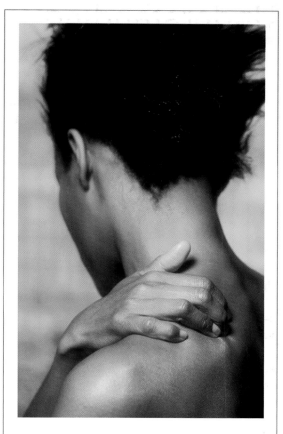

HOW OFTEN YOU SHOULD TREAT THE AREA

1 Massage each relevant muscle daily.

2 Work on removing trigger points every 2 to 3 days.

3 Stretch each relevant muscle twice a day. Continue this treatment for two weeks or until the pain has gone, whichever comes first.

IMPORTANT: If the muscle you are working feels no better—or has got worse—after two weeks, visit your doctor to rule out any underlying medical causes.

Pelvic muscles and pain

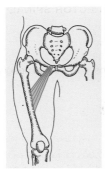

LOCATION
The anatomical location of the Adductor longus muscle (above).

AREA OF PAIN
The extent of pain referral originating from the Adductor longus (right).

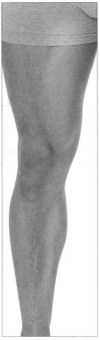

CAUSE OF PAIN: **ADDUCTOR LONGUS**

One end of this muscle is anchored to the side of the pubic bone; the other is attached to the inside of the thighbone (femur). When this muscle contracts, it draws your leg in from the side (adduction) and helps raise your thigh to the front.

Tightness and restriction can result from direct strain, overload, or injuries from splits-type motions (e.g. slipping with your legs splayed out while ice skating or skiing).

WHAT TO AVOID:

- Overstretching or bouncing when attempting the splits.
- Sitting with one leg crossed over the other, as this shortens the muscles on the upper leg and can lead to restriction and trigger-point formation.
- Prolonged contraction (adduction) of this muscle, e.g. during horseback riding. After dismounting, make sure you stretch the muscle out.

→ *see pages 106–7 for stretching and toning exercises*

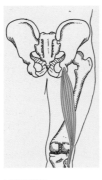

LOCATION
The anatomical location of the Biceps femoris muscle (above).

AREA OF PAIN
The extent of pain referral originating from the Biceps femoris muscle (right).

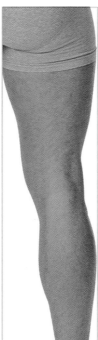

CAUSE OF PAIN:
BICEPS FEMORIS (HAMSTRINGS)

Part of the hamstrings group, this muscle is anchored to the bottom of the pelvis via the "sit bone" (ischial tuberosity) and to the back of the thighbone (femur). The other end attaches to the lower leg bone (fibula). When this muscle contracts, it bends your leg and pulls your thigh backward (hip extension). It also helps rotate your thigh outward when the knee is bent.

Restriction can result from direct trauma or prolonged shortening (e.g. too much sitting down). Keep this muscle stretched, especially after sports.

WHAT TO AVOID:

- Prolonged sitting in chairs that push into the backs of your thighs (e.g. deck chairs). Choose those with rounded, well-padded front edges.
- Failing to warm up thoroughly before participating in sports that involve running and jumping.

→ *see pages 108–9 for stretching and toning exercises*

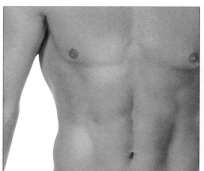

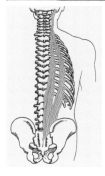

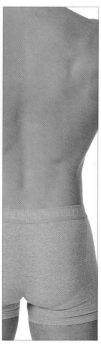

LOCATION
The anatomical location of the Erector spinae muscles (left).

AREA OF PAIN
The extent of pain referral originating from the Erector spinae muscles (above and right).

CAUSE OF PAIN: **ERECTOR SPINAE**

This group consists primarily of the Longissimus thoracis, Iliocostalis, and Spinalis muscles, and runs from the skull down to the base of the spine (sacrum). Each end of this group has the ability to move the spine, so the usual designation of "anchor-and-attachment point" is not easy to define. The primary muscles are connected to the 7th to 19th spinal vertebrae, the rear ribs, the sacrum, and the back ridge of the pelvis. When one side of this muscle contracts, it helps you bend to the side. When both sides contract, they help you lean backward and arch your back.

Tightness and restriction can result from direct trauma (tearing or straining of the muscle) and chronic overload (being worked too hard, for too long, too often, or any combination of these).

WHAT TO AVOID:
- Lifting objects without bending your knees.
- Sitting in the same position for long periods of time. Take breaks, get up, and move around.
- Sudden or awkward bending or twisting movements.
- Sleeping on very soft mattresses.

→ *see pages 110–115 for stretching and toning exercises*

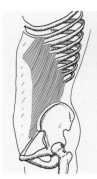

LOCATION
The anatomical location of the External oblique muscle (above).

AREA OF PAIN
The extent of pain referral originating from the External oblique muscle (right).

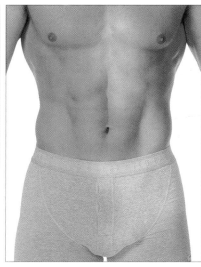

CAUSE OF PAIN: **EXTERNAL OBLIQUE**

This muscle covers the front side of the abdominal area and is anchored to the outer parts of the eight lowest ribs. Its other end attaches along the top front edge of the pelvis and joins to the connective tissue of the abdominal wall (abdominal aponeurosis). When this muscle contracts on one side, it helps you bend to that side and also rotates your spine. When both sides contract, this helps you bend your torso forward (e.g. when doing sit-ups). This muscle also helps support your internal organs.

Tightness and restriction can result from direct strain, chronic or acute overload (being worked too hard, for too long, too often, or any combination of these). Abdominal surgery can also cause dysfunction to these muscles (e.g. trigger points may form in, and around, post-surgical appendicitis scar tissue).

WHAT TO AVOID:
- Slouching when standing up or sitting down.
- Twisting your body when carrying heavy or awkward loads.

→ *see pages 116–118 for stretching and toning exercises*

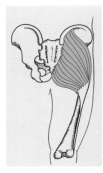

LOCATION
The anatomical location of the Gluteus maximus muscle (above).

AREA OF PAIN
The extent of pain referral originating from the Gluteus maximus muscle (right).

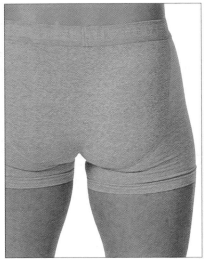

CAUSE OF PAIN: **GLUTEUS MAXIMUS**

This muscle has a complicated set of anchor points that cover the pelvis (posterior iliac crest), the sacrum, the coccyx, the ligament that runs from the sacrum to the pelvis, and the connective tissue on the Gluteus medius. The other end attaches to the thighbone and to the connective tissue (iliotibial band) that binds to the Tensor fasciae latae and runs down the outside of the thigh. When this muscle contracts, it pulls your thigh backward (extension) and turns your leg out, and it helps you raise your leg to the side.

Tightness and restriction can result from direct injury (e.g. from a fall) or prolonged compression. Keep this muscle stretched and supple, especially after strenuous activity and sports.

WHAT TO AVOID:

- Leaning over repeatedly when moving a heavy object (e.g. loading the trunk of a car).
- Sitting in the same position for long periods at a time. Get up regularly and move around.
- Sitting on hard objects (e.g. your wallet in your back pocket).
- Failing to stretch after swimming or power-lifting.

→ *see pages 119–120 for stretching and toning exercises*

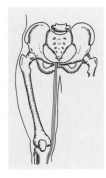

LOCATION
The anatomical location of the Gracilis muscle (above).

AREA OF PAIN
The extent of pain referral originating from the Gracilis muscle (right).

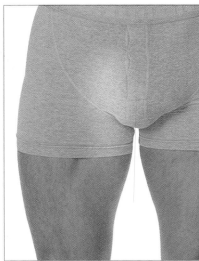

CAUSE OF PAIN: **GRACILIS**

This muscle is anchored to the lower ridge of the upper pubic bone. Its other end is attached to the upper inside surface of the shinbone (tibia). When it contracts, it draws your leg in from the side (adduction) and helps rotate your lower leg inward when your knee is bent.

Tightness and restriction can result from direct strain, overload, or injuries from splits-type motions (e.g. slipping with your legs splayed out while ice skating or skiing).

WHAT TO AVOID:

- Overstretching or bouncing when you do splits.
- Sitting with one leg crossed over the other, as this shortens the muscles on the upper leg and can lead to restriction and trigger-point formation.
- Prolonged contraction (adduction) of this muscle, e.g. during horseback riding. After dismounting, make sure you stretch the muscle out.

→ *see pages 106–7 for stretching and toning exercises*

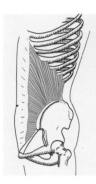

LOCATION
The anatomical location of the Internal oblique muscle (above).

AREA OF PAIN
The extent of pain referral originating from the Internal oblique muscle (right).

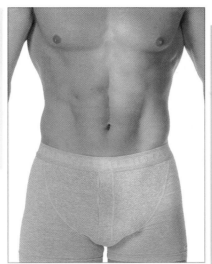

CAUSE OF PAIN: **INTERNAL OBLIQUE**

Lying directly underneath the External oblique, this muscle is anchored to the front two-thirds of the upper pelvis (anterior iliac crest), the connective tissue in the lower back (lumbar fascia), and to a ligament (inguinal ligament) that runs from the prominent bone at the front of the hips to the edge of the pubic bone. The opposite end of this fan-like muscle is attached to the last three or four ribs and the connective tissue that extends from the ribs down to the pubic bone. When this muscle contracts on one side, it helps you bend to that side and rotates your spine. When both sides contract, this bends your torso forward (e.g. for sit-ups). It also helps support the internal organs.

Shortening and restriction can result from direct strain and chronic or acute overload. Abdominal surgery can also cause dysfunction (e.g. trigger points may form in, and around post-surgical appendicitis scar tissue).

WHAT TO AVOID:
• Slouching when standing up or sitting down.
• Twisting your body when carrying heavy or awkward loads.

→ *see pages 116–118 for stretching and toning exercises*

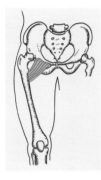

LOCATION
The anatomical location of the Pectineus muscle (above).

AREA OF PAIN
The extent of pain referral originating from the Pectineus muscle (right).

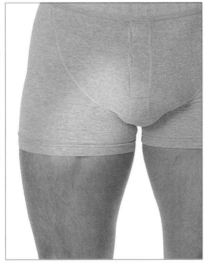

CAUSE OF PAIN: **PECTINEUS**

This muscle is anchored to the lower part of the bony ridge at the front of the pelvis (superior pubic ramus). Its opposite end is attached to the upper inside surface of the thighbone (femur). When this muscle contracts, it draws your leg in from the side (adduction), it also helps lift your thigh up to the front or helps you perform a combination of these movements.

Shortening and restriction can result from direct strain, overload, or injuries from splits-type motions (e.g. slipping with your legs splayed out while ice skating or skiing).

WHAT TO AVOID:
• Overstretching or bouncing when you do splits.
• Sitting with one leg crossed over the other, as this shortens the muscles on the upper leg and can lead to restriction and trigger-point formation.
• Prolonged contraction (adduction) of this muscle, e.g. during horseback riding. After dismounting, make sure you stretch the muscle out.

→ *see pages 106–7 for stretching and toning exercises*

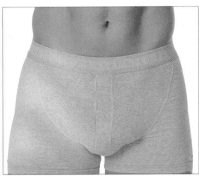

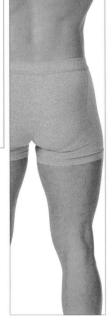

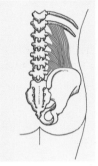

LOCATION
The anatomical location of the Quadratus lumborum muscle (left).

AREA OF PAIN
The extent of pain referral originating from the Quadratus lumborum muscle (above and right).

CAUSE OF PAIN: **QUADRATUS LUMBORUM**

This muscle is anchored to the rear upper pelvic curve (posterior iliac crest) and to a ligament (iliolumbar) running between the last spinal vertebrae and the iliac crest. Its opposite end is attached to the last rib and to bony attachments on the 20th to 23rd spinal vertebrae. When this muscle contracts on one side, it helps you bend to that side. When both sides contract, they help you lean backward. This muscle is also an important stabilizer of the spine.

WHAT TO AVOID:

- Twisting your body to lift awkward loads.
- Repetitive bending and twisting movements (e.g. digging).
- Twisting or bending to the side when you lift heavy objects.
- Leaning backward (e.g. to paint the ceiling) for a prolonged period of time. Have regular breaks.
- Lifting heavy objects without bending your knees.
- Sleeping on sagging mattresses that do not support your back.
- Sitting on a hard object (e.g. a wallet inside your back pocket).
- Running or jogging on unevenly sloping surfaces.

→ *see pages 142–4 for stretching and toning exercises*

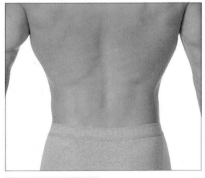

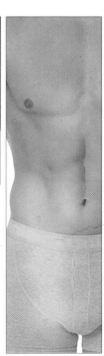

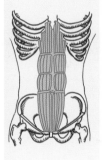

LOCATION
The anatomical location of the Rectus abdominis muscle (left).

AREA OF PAIN
The extent of pain referral originating from the Rectus abdominis muscle (above and right).

CAUSE OF PAIN: **RECTUS ABDOMINIS**

This muscle is anchored along the top edge of the pubic bone. Its other end is attached to the cartilage of the 5th, 6th, and 7th ribs at the joins with the breastbone and to the small pointed bone at the base of the breastbone. When this muscle contracts, it flexes your spine and pelvis forward (e.g. to curl up into a ball). It also helps support your internal organs.

Tightness and restriction can result from direct strain, poor posture, trauma (e.g. surgery), and chronic overload (being worked too hard, for too long, too often, or any combination of these). Keep this muscle stretched and supple, especially after strenuous activity and sports.

WHAT TO AVOID:

- Slouching when sitting down for long periods of time (e.g. while typing, writing, or reading).

→ *see page 145 for stretching and toning exercises*

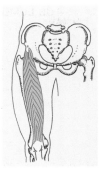

LOCATION
The anatomical location of the Rectus femoris muscle (above).

AREA OF PAIN
The extent of pain referral originating from the Rectus femoris muscle (right).

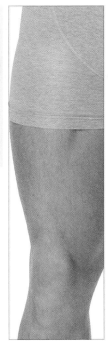

CAUSE OF PAIN: **RECTUS FEMORIS**

This muscle is anchored just below the prominent bone at the front of the hips (anterior superior iliac spine) and to a point just on the other side of it (posterior brim of the acetabulum). The opposite end attaches to the upper portion of the kneecap (patella) and the front of the upper shinbone (tibia) via a ligament sheath. Contraction of this muscle allows you to straighten your leg and helps raise your thigh to the front.

Tightness and restriction can result from direct trauma, sudden or rapid lengthening, and chronic overload (being worked too hard, for too long, too often, or any combination of these). Keep this muscle stretched and supple, especially after strenuous activity or sport.

WHAT TO AVOID:
- Sitting with one leg folded underneath you.
- Deep squatting movements if you have injured this muscle.
- Long periods of inactivity on long train or plane journeys. Get up regularly to move around.

→ **see pages 147–8 for stretching and toning exercises**

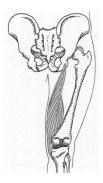 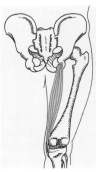

LOCATION
The anatomical location of the Semimembranosus (above left) and Semitendinosus muscles (above right).

AREA OF PAIN
Pain referred from the Semimembranosus and Semitendinosus muscles extends over the same area (right).

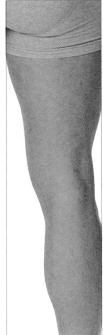

CAUSE OF PAIN: **SEMIMEMBRANOSUS AND SEMITENDINOSUS (HAMSTRINGS)**

Part of the hamstrings group, these muscles are anchored to the bottom of the pelvis via the "sit bone" (ischial tuberosity). The other ends attach to the upper shinbone (tibia)—the Semimembranosus attaches at the back, and the Semitendinosus on the inside surface. When these muscles contract, they bend your leg at the knee (flexion) and help rotate your thigh toward your body and pull it back (extension).

Tightness and restriction can result from direct trauma or prolonged shortening (e.g. from too much sitting down). Keep these muscles stretched and supple, especially after strenuous activity or sport.

WHAT TO AVOID:
- Prolonged sitting in chairs with frames that push into the backs of your thighs (e.g. deck chairs). Choose those with rounded, well-padded front edges.
- Participating in sports that involve running and jumping without thoroughly warming up your legs beforehand.

→ **see pages 108–9 for stretching and toning exercises**

Shoulder muscles and pain

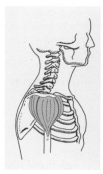

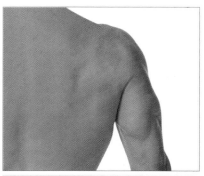

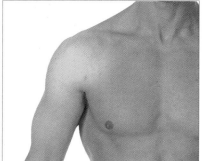

LOCATION
The anatomical location of the Deltoid muscle (above).

AREA OF PAIN
The extent of pain referral originating from the Deltoid muscle (right).

CAUSE OF PAIN: **DELTOID**

This muscle is made up of three heads: the anterior, medial, and posterior. The anterior head is anchored to the outer third of the collarbone (clavicle); the medial head to the curved finger of bone (acromion) on the outside of the shoulder blade (scapula); and the posterior head is anchored to the bony ridge that runs along the upper-third of the shoulder blade. The opposite ends of all three heads connect about halfway down the outside surface of the upper arm bone (humerus). This muscle helps lift your arm away from your side (abduction), to the front (flexion), and behind you (extension), and aids in pulling it across your chest.

   Although not involved in specific distortions, the Deltoid can play a significant role in shoulder pain. The exercises that stretch the Pectoralis major and Middle trapezius muscles also help to stretch the Deltoid.

→ *the exercises on pages 136 and 138 also help to stretch the Deltoid*

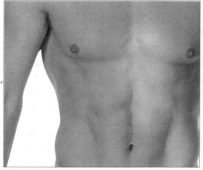

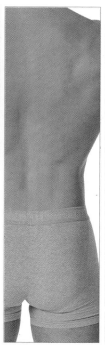

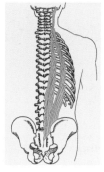

LOCATION
The anatomical location of the Erector spinae muscle group (left).

AREA OF PAIN
The extent of pain referral originating from the Erector spinae muscle group (above and right).

CAUSE OF PAIN: **ERECTOR SPINAE**

This group consists primarily of the Longissimus thoracis, Iliocostalis, and Spinalis muscles, and runs from the skull down to the base of the spine (sacrum). Each end of this group has the ability to move the spine, so the usual designation of "anchor-and-attachment point" is not easy to define. The primary muscles are connected to the 7th to 19th spinal vertebrae, the rear ribs, the sacrum, and the back ridge of the pelvis. When one side of this muscle contracts, it helps you bend to the side. When both sides contract, they help you lean backward and arch your back.

   Tightness and restriction can result from direct trauma (tearing or straining of the muscle) and chronic overload (being worked too hard, for too long, too often, or any combination of these).

WHAT TO AVOID:
- Lifting objects without bending your knees.
- Sitting in the same position for long periods of time. Take breaks, get up, and move around.
- Sudden or awkward bending or twisting movements.
- Sleeping on very soft mattresses.

→ *see pages 110–115 for stretching and toning exercises*

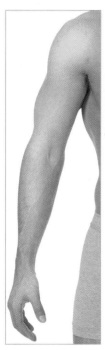
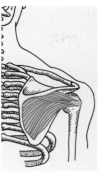
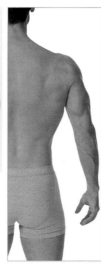

LOCATION
The anatomical location of the Infraspinatus muscle (above).

AREA OF PAIN
The extent of pain referral originating from the Infraspinatus muscle (left and above).

CAUSE OF PAIN: **INFRASPINATUS**

This muscle is anchored to the bottom two-thirds of the shoulder blade (scapula) near its inside edge. Its other end is attached to the back portion of the upper arm bone (humerus). The major function of this muscle is to turn your arm outward (external rotation), but it also stabilizes the head of your arm bone within its shoulder socket.

Although tightness and restriction can result from direct injury (e.g. reaching back to grab the railing to avoid tripping down steps or having your arm jerked back e.g. wrestling or martial arts moves), this muscle is more commonly injured through chronic overload (being worked too hard, for too long, too often, or any combination of these). Keep it stretched and supple, especially after strenuous activity or sport.

WHAT TO AVOID:
• Positions and surroundings that can cause repetitive strain injury (RSI), e.g. repeatedly reaching out behind you.

→ *see pages 126–7 for stretching and toning exercises*

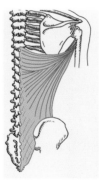
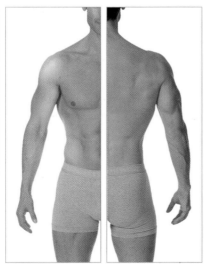

LOCATION
The anatomical location of the Latissimus dorsi muscle (above).

AREA OF PAIN
The extent of pain referral originating from the Latissimus dorsi muscle (right).

CAUSE OF PAIN: **LATISSIMUS DORSI**

This muscle is anchored to the last 11 bones in the spine, the flat bone at the base of the spine (sacrum), the top of the pelvis, and the four lower ribs. Its other end is attached to the top of the arm bone (humerus), just below the shoulder. Its function is to draw your arm back and in toward your body (extension and adduction) and help rotate it inward. The upper fibers of this muscle can also draw your shoulder blade down (depression) and in (retraction).

Tightness and restriction can result from repetitive and sustained reaching forward and up movements; chronic overload and trauma; reaching overhead with heavy weights; or catching fast-moving balls at full stretch.

WHAT TO AVOID:
• Continuous and repetitive movements (e.g. painting high walls, reaching up to clean windows, plastering). Take regular breaks, shift positions, and change hands.
• Moving heavy and/or awkward loads.

→ *see pages 128–9 for stretching and toning exercises*

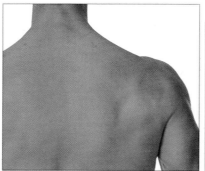

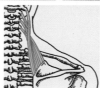

LOCATION
The anatomical location of the Levator scapulae muscle (right).

AREA OF PAIN
The extent of pain referral originating from the Levator scapulae muscle (above).

CAUSE OF PAIN: **LEVATOR SCAPULAE**

This muscle is anchored to the sides of the upper four neck vertebrae. Its other end is fixed to the upper inside edge of the shoulder blade (scapula). When it contracts, it helps lift your shoulder, rotates your neck on that side, or does both together.

Tightness and restriction can result from neck injuries (e.g. whiplash) or chronic overload (being used too hard, for too long, too often, or a combination of these). Keep this muscle stretched and supple, especially after strenuous activity.

WHAT TO AVOID:

- Prolonged contraction of the neck and shoulder (e.g. from cradling the telephone handset between your shoulder and ear).
- Prolonged elevation positions that leave shoulders tight and hunched. Ensure that chair armrests are not excessively high.
- Carrying heavy shoulder bags.
- Prolonged rotation of the neck (e.g. from keeping your head turned at an angle while working at your computer).
- Tight, narrow bra straps, as they can cause trigger points.

→ **see pages 130–131 for stretching and toning exercises**

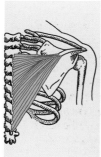

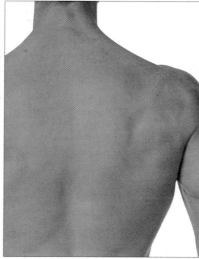

LOCATION
The anatomical location of the Lower trapezius muscle (above).

AREA OF PAIN
The extent of pain referral originating from the Lower trapezius muscle (right).

CAUSE OF PAIN: **LOWER TRAPEZIUS**

This muscle is anchored to the prominent bones on the backs of the 12th to 20th spinal vertebrae. Its other end is attached to the inner third of the horizontal bony ridge that runs across the shoulder blade (scapula). Contraction of this muscle pulls your scapula toward your spine (retraction), rotates it outward, and help lift your arm away from your body (abduction).

Tightness and restriction can result from repetitive and constant bending over or reaching forward movements while sitting down.

WHAT TO AVOID:

- Sitting at a desk under which you cannot comfortably slide your knees. This will make leaning, reaching, or stretching forward necessary while you work.

→ **see pages 134–5 for stretching and toning exercises**

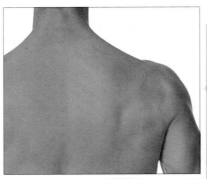

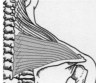

LOCATION
The anatomical location of the Middle trapezius muscle (right).

AREA OF PAIN
The extent of pain referral originating from the Middle trapezius muscle (above).

CAUSE OF PAIN: **MIDDLE TRAPEZIUS**

This muscle is anchored to the prominent bones on the backs of the 6th to 11th spinal vertebrae. The other end of this muscle is attached to the upper portion of the shoulder blade. The primary function of this muscle is to pull your shoulder blade (scapula) toward your spine. It also helps rotate it outward (abduction).

Tightness and restriction can result from chronic overload, direct strain, poor posture, and an already tight or restricted Pectoralis major muscle (see below).

WHAT TO AVOID:

- Sitting down for long periods of time with rounded shoulders (e.g. while typing, writing, or reading). Take breaks, get up, and move around.
- Holding your arms in front of you for a prolonged period of time.
- Tightly gripping the top of the steering wheel of your car for long periods of time, as this rounds the shoulders and can also chronically overload this muscle.

→ **see pages 136–7 for *stretching and toning exercises***

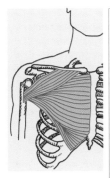

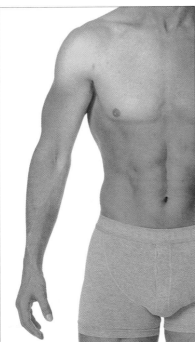

LOCATION
The anatomical location of the Pectoralis major muscle (above).

AREA OF PAIN
The extent of pain referral originating from the Pectoralis major muscle (right).

CAUSE OF PAIN: **PECTORALIS MAJOR**

This muscle group is made up of three layers: the clavicular, sternal, and costal. The clavicular head is fastened to the half of the collarbone (clavicle) closest to the breastbone; the sternal head is attached to the breastbone (sternum); and the costal head is anchored to parts of the 2nd to 6th or 7th ribs by the breastbone. The other end of this muscle group connects to the top of the arm bone (humerus). This muscle group's major function is to draw your arms to your sides (mainly the sternal head), across your chest, rotate your arms inward (internal rotation), or any combination of these.

Tightness and restriction result from direct injury, poor postural habits (e.g. slouching), or chronic overload (being worked too hard, for too long, too often, or any combination of these). Keep this group of muscles stretched and supple, especially after strenuous activity.

WHAT TO AVOID:

- Sitting hunched forward with rounded shoulders for long periods of time (i.e. typing, writing, or reading).

→ **see pages 138–9 for *stretching and toning exercises***

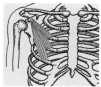

LOCATION
The anatomical location of the Pectoralis minor muscle (above).

AREA OF PAIN
The extent of pain referral originating from the Pectoralis minor muscle (right).

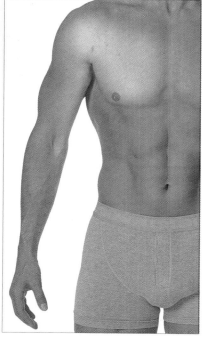

CAUSE OF PAIN: **PECTORALIS MINOR**

This muscle is anchored to the outer surface of the 3rd to 5th ribs. Its other end is attached to a bony prominence toward the top outside corner of the shoulder blade (coracoid process). Contraction of this muscle simultaneously pulls the upper outside edge of your shoulder blade forward, downward, and inward.

Tightness and restriction can result from direct strain and poor posture. Keep this muscle stretched and supple, especially after strenuous activity and sports.

WHAT TO AVOID:

- Sitting down for long periods of time with rounded shoulders (e.g. when typing, writing, or reading).
- Prolonged pressure on this muscle area (e.g. from tightly strapping a backpack across the shoulders).

→ *see pages 138–9 for stretching and toning exercises*

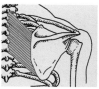

LOCATION
The anatomical location of the Rhomboid muscles (above).

AREA OF PAIN
The extent of pain referral originating in the Rhomboid muscles (right).

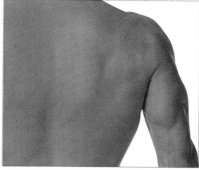

CAUSE OF PAIN: **RHOMBOIDS**

These two muscles (rhomboideus major and minor) are anchored to the prominent bones on the backs of the 7th to 12th spinal vertebrae. The opposite ends of these muscles attach to the inner edge of the shoulder blade. When they contract, they pull your shoulder blades toward your spine, while their lower portions rotate your shoulder blades inward (adduction).

Tightness and restriction can result from direct strain, poor posture (especially when sitting down), and muscular weakness, often caused by tightness in the Pectoralis major muscles, see page 107).

WHAT TO AVOID:

- Sitting down for long periods of time with rounded shoulders (e.g. when typing, writing, or reading). Have breaks, get up, and move around.

→ *see pages 136–7 for stretching and toning exercises*

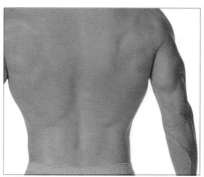

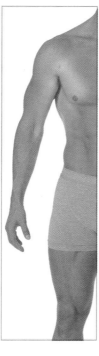

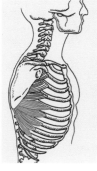

LOCATION
The anatomical location of the Serratus anterior muscle (left).

AREA OF PAIN
The extent of pain referral originating from the Serratus anterior muscle (above and right).

CAUSE OF PAIN: **SERRATUS ANTERIOR**

This muscle is anchored to the first eight or nine ribs. Its other end is attached along the back of the inner edge of the shoulder blade closest to the spine. Its function is to pull your shoulder blade (scapula) sideways and away from the spine (protraction), rotate your scapula (abduction), and elevate your shoulder (especially the middle portion of this muscle).

Tightness and restriction can result from intense physical activity like running (both sprinting and long distance), lifting heavy overhead weights (e.g. during shoulder presses), bench-presses, push-ups, and violent coughing fits. Keep this muscle stretched and supple, especially after strenuous activity and sports.

➜ *see page 152 for stretching and toning exercises*

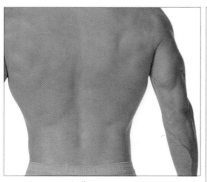

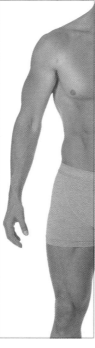

LOCATION
The anatomical location of the Serratus anterior muscle (left).

AREA OF PAIN
The extent of pain referral originating from the Serratus anterior muscle (above and right).

CAUSE OF PAIN:
SERRATUS ANTERIOR (LOWER FIBERS)

The lower and strongest portion of this muscle is anchored to the 4th or 5th to the 8th or 9th ribs. Its other end is attached to the bottom angle (costal surface) of the shoulder blade. This muscle rotates your shoulder blade outward (abduction) and its middle portion helps raise your shoulder.

Tightness and restriction can result from intense physical activity like running (both sprinting and long distance), lifting heavy overhead weights (e.g. during shoulder presses), bench-presses, push-ups, and violent coughing fits. Keep this muscle stretched and supple, especially after strenuous activity and sports.

➜ *see pages 152 for stretching and toning exercises*

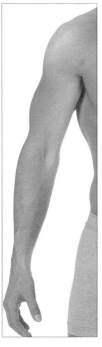
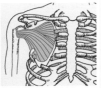
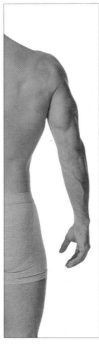

LOCATION
The anatomical location of the Subscapularis muscle (above).

AREA OF PAIN
The extent of pain referral originating from the Subscapularis muscle (left and right).

CAUSE OF PAIN: **SUBSCAPULARIS**

This muscle is anchored to the flat internal surface of the shoulder blade (subscapular fossa). Its other end is attached to the upper front side of the arm bone and shoulder joint. When this muscle contracts, it rotates your arm inward and helps draw your arm into your side (adduction).

Tightness and restriction can result from direct strain and chronic overload (e.g. reaching back with your arm to brace yourself against a fall or throwing an object). Keep this muscle stretched and supple, especially after strenuous activity or sport.

WHAT TO AVOID:
- Failing to warm-up your shoulder muscles before participating in activities that involve throwing or swimming.

→ *see page 155 for stretching and toning exercises*

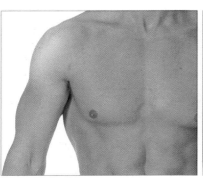
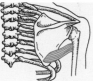
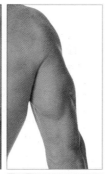
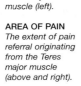
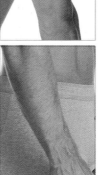

LOCATION
The anatomical location of the Teres major muscle (left).

AREA OF PAIN
The extent of pain referral originating from the Teres major muscle (above and right).

CAUSE OF PAIN: **TERES MAJOR**

This muscle is anchored to the bottom outside edge of the shoulder blade. Its other end attaches to the upper front part of the arm bone (lesser tubercule of the humerus). Contraction of this muscle helps pull your arm in to your side, rotate it inward, and pull it back.

Tightness and restriction can result from chronic overload (e.g. driving a motor vehicle with heavy steering).

WHAT TO AVOID:
- Driving vehicles not fitted with power-steering.

→ *see pages 128–9 for stretching and toning exercises*

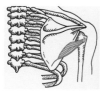

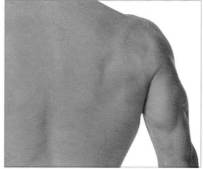

LOCATION
The anatomical location of the Teres minor muscle (above).

AREA OF PAIN
The extent of pain referral originating from the Teres minor muscle (right).

CAUSE OF PAIN: **TERES MINOR**

This muscle is anchored to the middle outside edge of the shoulder blade nearest to the arm bone. Its other end attaches to the upper portion of the back of the arm bone (humerus), just under the attachment point for the Infraspinatus (see page 105). Contraction of the Teres minor turns your arm outward (external rotation) and helps stabilize the arm bone in the shoulder socket.

Tightness and restriction can result from direct injury (e.g. reaching back to grab the railing when tripping down steps or having your arm jerked back e.g. wrestling or martial arts) and chronic overload (being worked too hard, for too long, too often, or any combination of these). Keep this muscle stretched and supple, especially after strenuous activity and sports.

WHAT TO AVOID:

- Positions and surroundings that cause you to frequently reach out behind you for a prolonged period of time.

→ **see pages 126–7 for stretching and toning exercises**

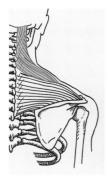

LOCATION
The anatomical location of the Upper trapezius muscle (above).

AREA OF PAIN
The extent of pain referral originating from the Upper trapezius muscle (right).

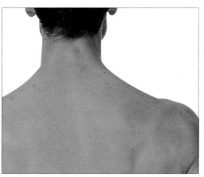

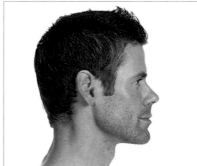

CAUSE OF PAIN: **UPPER TRAPEZIUS**

This muscle is anchored to the base of the skull (occiput) and to the upper five neck vertebrae. Its other end is attached to the outer third of the collarbone (clavicle). When this muscle contracts on one side, it elevates the shoulder, rotates it upward (abduction), and/or bends your neck toward that shoulder. When both sides contract, they push your head and neck forward against resistance.

Tightness and restriction can result from whiplash-type injuries or chronic overload (being worked too hard, for too long, too often, or a combination of these). Keep this muscle stretched and supple, particularly after strenuous activities and sport.

WHAT TO AVOID:

- Prolonged contraction of the neck and shoulder (e.g. cradling a telephone handset between your ear and shoulder or turning your head at an angle to look at your computer).
- Sitting in chairs with high armrests over long periods of time.
- Carrying heavy shoulder bags.
- Tight, narrow bra straps, as these can cause trigger points.

→ **see pages 156–7 for stretching and toning exercises**

Head and neck muscles and pain

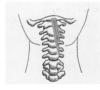

LOCATION
The anatomical location of the Longus capitis muscle (above).

AREA OF PAIN
The extent of pain referral originating from the Longus capitis muscle (right).

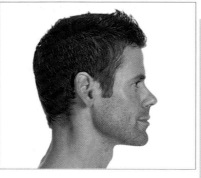

CAUTION
It is not advisable to massage and press into the front of your neck and throat area unless you have had the necessary therapeutic training allowing you to do so safely. Instead, use the stretching exercises to lengthen the Longus capitis muscle.

CAUSE OF PAIN: **LONGUS CAPITIS**

This muscle is anchored to the front sides of the 3rd to 5th neck vertebrae. Its other end attaches underneath the bone at the back of the head (occipital bone). When this muscle contracts, it rotates your head and helps bend it forward.

This muscle is often damaged in whiplash injuries. As tightness increases, the discs between each neck vertebra push together, in turn forcing the discs between the bones into the nerves at the back of the neck. This causes increased pain.

→ *see pages 132–3 for stretching and toning exercises*

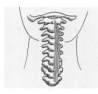

LOCATION
The anatomical location of the Longus colli muscle (above).

AREA OF PAIN
The extent of pain referral originating in the Longus colli muscle (right).

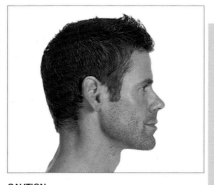

CAUTION
It is not advisable to massage and press into the front of your neck and throat area unless you have had the necessary therapeutic training allowing you to do so safely. Instead, use the stretching exercises to lengthen the Longus colli muscle.

CAUSE OF PAIN: **LONGUS COLLI**

This muscle is split into three parts: vertical, upper oblique, and lower oblique. The vertical part is anchored to the middle of the 5th to 10th vertebrae and connects to the 2nd to 4th vertebrae in the front of the neck. Its upper oblique portion is anchored to the front sides of the 3rd to 5th neck vertebrae and attaches to a prominent bone (tubercule) on the top vertebrae in the neck. The lower oblique portion is anchored to the front of the first three neck vertebrae and attaches to the front sides of the 5th and 6th vertebrae in the neck. Contraction of this muscle rotates your head and helps you bend your neck forward. Contraction on one side helps you bend your head to that side.

There are no specific activities that you need to avoid to protect the Longus colli. But keep it stretched and supple, especially after strenuous activity or sports.

→ *see pages 132–3 for stretching and toning exercises*

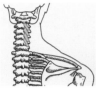

LOCATION
The anatomical location of the Multifidi muscles (above).

AREA OF PAIN
The extent of pain referral originating from the Multifidi muscles (right).

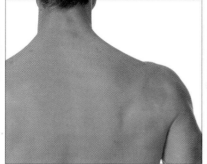

CAUSE OF PAIN: **MULTIFIDI (UPPER SECTION)**

These muscles run down the length of your spine. Their upper sections are anchored to the prominent bones at the back of the 2nd to 5th neck vertebrae. The opposite ends of these muscles are attached to the 4th to 7th bones in the neck. When these muscles contract, they help you bend to that side and help rotate your spine toward the opposite side.

Shortening and restriction result from direct injury or chronic overload. This can be seen often in people who cycle or ride motorcycles: in order to look straight ahead, they need to tilt their heads back while they bend forward. Stretch out these muscles after cycling or riding motorcycles for long periods.

WHAT TO AVOID:

- Prolonged hyper-extension (pulling back) of the head (e.g. while painting a high wall or ceiling). Have regular breaks and don't keep your neck fixed in this position for long periods of time.
- Prolonged neck contraction (e.g. cradling the telephone between your ear and shoulder). Switch sides regularly.
- Head-circling exercises in which you tilt your head back.

→ *see pages 153–4 for stretching and toning exercises*

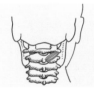

LOCATION
The anatomical location of the Obliquus capitis inferior muscle (above).

AREA OF PAIN
The extent of pain referral originating from the Obliquus capitis inferior muscle (right).

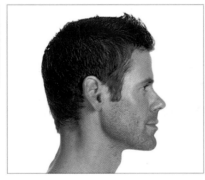

CAUSE OF PAIN: **OBLIQUUS CAPITIS INFERIOR**

This muscle is anchored to the middle of the 2nd vertebra in the neck, while the opposite end attaches to the side of the top vertebra in the neck. When this muscle contracts, it helps rotate your head to that side.

Tightness and restriction can result from chronic overload (being worked too hard, for too long, too often, or a combination of these).

WHAT TO AVOID:

- Prolonged hyper-extension (pulling back) of the head (e.g. while painting a ceiling, or sitting too close to the screen at the movies). Have regular breaks and don't keep your neck fixed in this position for long periods of time.
- Prolonged neck rotation (e.g. working at a computer screen with your neck turned at an angle).

→ *see page 146 for stretching and toning exercises*

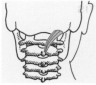

LOCATION
The anatomical location of the Rectus capitis posterior major muscle (above).

AREA OF PAIN
The extent of pain referral originating from the Rectus capitis posterior major muscle (right).

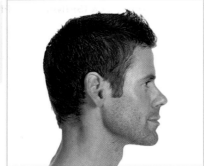

CAUSE OF PAIN:
RECTUS CAPITIS POSTERIOR MAJOR

This muscle is anchored to the prominent bone on the back of the 2nd vertebra of the neck. The other end attaches to the bony ridge on the back of the skull (occipital ridge). Contraction of this muscle helps rotate your head and assists side tilt.

Tightness can results from chronic overload (being worked too hard, for too long, too often, or a combination of these).

WHAT TO AVOID:
- Prolonged hyper-extension (pulling back) of the head (e.g. while painting a ceiling or sitting too close to the screen at the movies). Have regular breaks and don't keep your neck fixed in this position for long periods of time.
- Prolonged neck rotation (e.g. working at a computer screen with your neck turned at an angle).
- Letting the back of your neck become chilled.

→ *see page 146 for stretching and toning exercises*

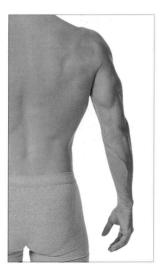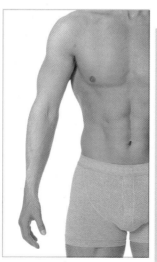

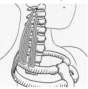

LOCATION
The anatomical location of the Scalenes muscle (left).

AREA OF PAIN
The extent of pain referral originating from the Scalenes muscle (above).

CAUSE OF PAIN: **SCALENES**

This group has four separate heads. The anterior head is anchored between the 3rd to 6th neck vertebrae and attached to the first rib. The Scalene medius is anchored to the 2nd to 7th vertebrae in the neck and attached to the side of the first rib. The Scalene minimus is anchored to the 6th or 7th neck vertebrae and attached to the first rib. The Scalene posterior is anchored to the 5th to 7th neck vertebrae and attached to the outside of the second and sometimes third rib. When these muscles contract on one side, they tilt your head sideways (lateral flexion). When they contract on both sides, they tilt your neck forward (neck flexion). They are also vital to your breathing.

Tightness and restriction can result from direct strain and chronic overload. Stretch these muscles after strenuous activity.

WHAT TO AVOID:
- Prolonged neck contractions (e.g. nestling a telephone between your ear and shoulder). Switch sides regularly.
- Sitting on chairs with raised armrests.

→ *see pages 149–50 for stretching and toning exercises*

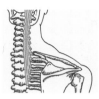

LOCATION
The anatomical location of the Semispinalis capitis muscle (above).

AREA OF PAIN
The extent of pain referral originating from the Semispinalis capitis muscle (right).

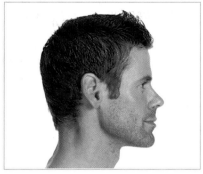

CAUSE OF PAIN: **SEMISPINALIS CAPITIS**

This muscle is anchored above the bony ridge at the base of the skull (occiput). Its other end is attached to the sides of the 3rd to 13th spinal vertebrae. When this muscle contracts, it helps tilt your head backward (extension).

Shortening and restriction can result from direct injury or chronic overload. This can be seen often in people who cycle or ride motorcycles: in order to look straight ahead, they need to tilt their heads back while they bend forward. Stretch out these muscles after cycling or riding motorcycles for long periods.

WHAT TO AVOID:

- Prolonged hyper-extension (pulling back) of the head (e.g. while painting a high wall or ceiling). Have regular breaks and don't keep your neck fixed in this position for long periods of time.
- Prolonged neck contraction (e.g. cradling the telephone between your ear and shoulder). Switch sides regularly.
- Head-circling exercises in which you tilt your head back.

➜ *see page 151 for stretching and toning exercises*

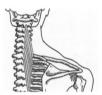

LOCATION
The anatomical location of the Semispinalis cervicis muscle (above).

AREA OF PAIN
The extent of pain referral originating from the Semispinalis cervicis muscle (right).

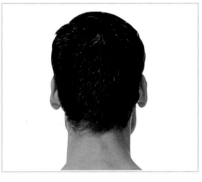

CAUSE OF PAIN: **SEMISPINALIS CERVICIS**

This muscle is anchored to the prominent bones of the 2nd to 5th neck vertebrae. Its other end attaches to the 8th to 14th spinal vertebrae. Contraction of this muscle helps tilt your head to the side (lateral flexion) and rotate your neck on the opposite side.

Shortening and restriction can result from direct injury or chronic overload. This can be seen often in people who cycle or ride motorcycles: in order to look straight ahead, they need to tilt their heads back while they bend forward. Stretch out these muscles after cycling or riding motorcycles for long periods.

WHAT TO AVOID:

- Prolonged hyper-extension (pulling back) of the head (e.g. while painting a high wall or ceiling). Have regular breaks and don't keep your neck fixed in this position for long periods of time.
- Prolonged neck contraction (e.g. cradling the telephone between your ear and shoulder). Switch sides regularly.
- Head-circling exercises in which you tilt your head back.

➜ *see page 151 for stretching and toning exercises*

LOCATION
The anatomical location of the Splenius capitis muscle (above).

AREA OF PAIN
The extent of pain referral originating from the Splenius capitis muscle (right).

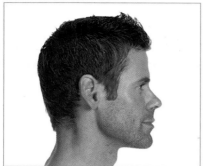

CAUSE OF PAIN: **SPLENIUS CAPITIS**

This muscle is anchored to the middle of the 3rd to 10th or 11th neck vertebrae. Its other end attaches to the bony protuberance at the bottom of the skull, just below and behind the ear (mastoid process), and to the bony ridge at the back of the skull (occipital ridge). Contraction of this muscle on one side helps rotate your head on that side. When this muscle contracts on both sides, it helps tilt your head back.

Tightness and restriction can result from direct strain or chronic overload. The Splenius capitis can also be damaged in whiplash-type injuries. Keep it stretched and supple, especially after strenuous activity.

WHAT TO AVOID:

- Prolonged hyper-extension (pulling back) of the head (e.g. while painting a high wall or ceiling). Have regular breaks and don't keep your neck in this fixed position for long periods of time.
- Prolonged neck rotation (e.g. working at a computer screen with your neck turned at an angle).

→ *see page 151 for stretching and toning exercises*

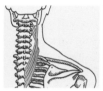

LOCATION
The anatomical location of the Splenius cervicis muscle (above).

AREA OF PAIN
The extent of pain referral originating from the Splenius cervicis muscle (right).

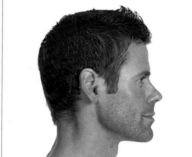

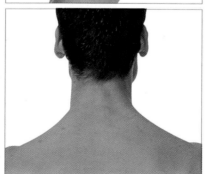

CAUSE OF PAIN: **SPLENIUS CERVICIS**

This muscle is anchored to the middle of the 10th to 13th spinal vertebrae. Its other end attaches to the sides of the upper 2 or 3 neck vertebrae. When this muscle contracts on one side, it helps bend and/or rotate your head in the same direction. When the muscle contracts on both sides, it helps tilt your neck back (the movement you do when looking up at something).

Tightness and restriction can result from direct strain or chronic overload (being worked too hard, for too long, too often, or any combination of these). This muscle can also be damaged in whiplash-type injuries. Keep it stretched and supple, especially after strenuous activity and sports.

WHAT TO AVOID:

- Prolonged hyper-extension (pulling back) of the head (e.g. while painting a high wall or ceiling). Have regular breaks and don't keep your neck in this fixed position for long periods of time.
- Prolonged neck rotation (e.g. working at a computer screen with your neck turned at an angle).

→ *see page 151 for stretching and toning exercises*

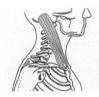

LOCATION
The anatomical location of the Sternocleidomastoid muscle (above).

AREA OF PAIN
The extent of pain referral originating from the Sternocleidomastoid muscle (right).

IMPORTANT
Pressing directly into this muscle when massaging can damage the carotid artery. Instead, tilt your head to the side you want to treat, rotate it slightly to loosen the muscle, then knead the muscle from the sides using your fingers and thumb.

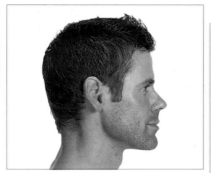

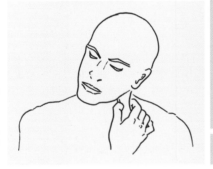

CAUSE OF PAIN: **STERNOCLEIDOMASTOID**

This muscle is made up of two heads. The sternal head is anchored to the outside edge of the breastbone. The clavicular head connects to the inner third of the collarbone (clavicle). The opposite ends of both heads attach to the bottom of the skull. When this muscle contracts on one side, it helps rotate and tilt your head to the opposite side. When both sides contract, they pull your head and neck forward.

Shortening and restriction result from whiplash-type injuries, direct trauma, or chronic overload.

WHAT TO AVOID:

- Slouching and sitting with your chin tucked into your chest.
- Pulling your head back for prolonged periods of time (e.g. looking up when painting a ceiling). Have regular breaks.
- Prolonged neck contractions (e.g. cradling the telephone between your ear and shoulder). Switch sides regularly.
- Pulling on your head with your hands when you perform sit-ups.
- Sleeping on your stomach with your head turned to one side.

→ *see pages 153–4 for stretching and toning exercises*

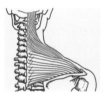

LOCATION
The anatomical location of the Upper trapezius muscle (above).

AREA OF PAIN
The extent of the region of discomfort caused by pain referral originating in the Upper trapezius muscle (right).

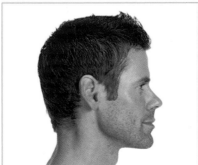

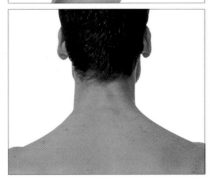

CAUSE OF PAIN: **UPPER TRAPEZIUS**

This muscle is anchored to the base of the skull and to the back of the first five vertebrae in the neck. Its other end attaches to the outer part of the collarbone (clavicle). When one side contracts, it elevates your shoulder and helps rotate it upward. It also allows you to bend your neck toward that shoulder, or do both simultaneously. When both sides contract, they help extend your neck forward against resistance.

Tightness and restriction result from whiplash-type injuries, during sport, or as the result of chronic overload. Keep this muscle stretched and supple, especially after strenuous activity.

WHAT TO AVOID:

- Prolonged neck contractions (e.g. cradling the telephone between your ear and shoulder). Switch sides regularly.
- Sitting in chairs with high armrests.
- Carrying heavy shoulder bags.
- Prolonged neck rotation (e.g. working at a computer screen with your neck turned at an angle).
- Wearing tight, narrow bra straps.

→ *see pages 156–7 for stretching and toning exercises*

Leg muscles and pain

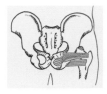

LOCATION
The anatomical location of the Deep rotators (above).

AREA OF PAIN
The extent of pain referral originating from the Deep rotators (right).

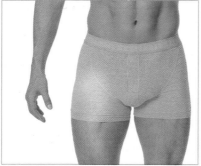

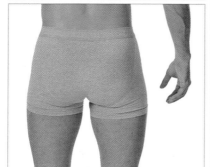

CAUSE OF PAIN: **DEEP ROTATORS**

These are the Superior and Inferior gemellus, Obturator internus and externus, and Quadratus femoris. Both gemellus muscles are anchored to the bottom of the pelvis via the "sit bone" (ischial tuberosity) and attached to the upper thighbone (greater trochanter). The Obturator internus is anchored to the bottom of the pelvis and to a membrane found there, and attached to the inside of the upper thighbone. The Obturator externus is anchored to the same pelvic membrane and attached to the upper thighbone. The Quadratus femoris is anchored to the ischial tuberosity and attached to the upper thighbone. When these muscles contract, they turn your leg outward (external rotation).

Tightness and restriction can result from direct injury and sudden or chronic overload twisting sideways to lift heavy objects). Keep this muscle stretched, especially after strenuous activity.

WHAT TO AVOID:
- Sitting with one leg folded underneath you.
- Long periods of inactivity on long train, plane, or car journeys. Get up regularly and walk around.

→ *see pages 140–1 for stretching and toning exercises*

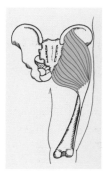

LOCATION
The anatomical location of the Gluteus maximus muscle (above).

AREA OF PAIN
The extent of pain referral originating from the Gluteus maximus muscle (right).

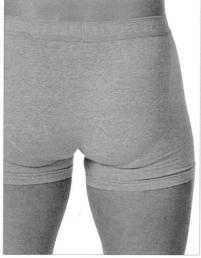

CAUSE OF PAIN: **GLUTEUS MAXIMUS**

This muscle has a complicated set of anchor points that cover the pelvis (posterior iliac crest), the sacrum, the coccyx, the ligament that runs from the sacrum to the pelvis, and the connective tissue on the Gluteus medius. The other end attaches to the thighbone and to the connective tissue (iliotibial band) that binds to the Tensor fasciae latae and runs down the outside of the thigh. When this muscle contracts, it pulls your thigh backward (extension) and turns your leg out, and it helps you raise your leg to the side.

Tightness and restriction can result from direct injury (e.g. from a fall) or prolonged compression. Keep this muscle stretched and supple, especially after strenuous activity and sports.

WHAT TO AVOID:
- Leaning over repeatedly when moving a heavy object (e.g. loading the trunk of a car).
- Sitting in the same position for long periods at a time. Get up regularly and move around.
- Sitting on hard objects (e.g. your wallet in your back pocket).
- Failing to stretch after swimming or power-lifting.

→ *see pages 119–120 for stretching and toning exercises*

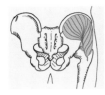

LOCATION
The anatomical location of the Gluteus medius muscle (left).

AREA OF PAIN
The extent of pain referral originating from the Gluteus medius muscle (right).

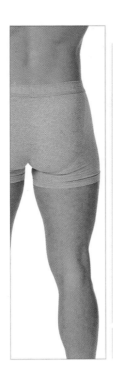

CAUSE OF PAIN: **GLUTEUS MEDIUS**

This muscle is anchored to the outside edge of the pelvis and to a thick sheet of connective tissue (gluteal aponeurosis) that covers it. Its other end attaches to a thick tendon that connects to the outside of the upper thighbone. When this muscle contracts, it moves your leg out and away from your body (abduction). It also helps turn your leg inward (internal rotation) and lift up your thigh.

Tightness and restriction can result from direct injury to the area (e.g. from a rugby tackle or a fall) and chronic overload (being used too hard, for too long, too often, or any combination of these). Keep this muscle stretched and supple, especially after strenuous activity and sports.

WHAT TO AVOID:

- Long periods of inactivity on long train, plane, or car journeys. Get up regularly and walk around.
- Sitting on hard objects (e.g. your wallet in your back pocket).

→ *see pages 121–3 for stretching and toning exercises*

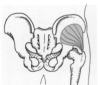

LOCATION
The anatomical location of the Gluteus minimus muscle (above).

AREA OF PAIN
The extent of pain referral originating from the Gluteus minimus muscle (right).

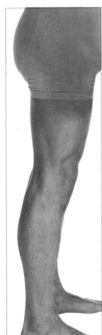 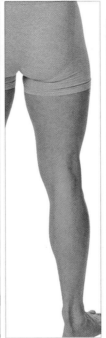

CAUSE OF PAIN: **GLUTEUS MINIMUS**

This muscle is anchored to the upper edge of the pelvis, just below the anchor point for the Gluteus medius muscle. Its other end attaches to the upper frontal portion of the thighbone. Contraction of this muscle helps move your leg out, away from your body (abduction), and turns it inward (internal rotation).

Tightness and restriction result from sudden trauma (e.g. a rugby tackle or a fall), chronic overload (being used too hard, for too long, too often, or any combination of these), or prolonged periods of inactivity. Keep this muscle stretched and supple, especially after strenuous activity and sports.

WHAT TO AVOID:

- Extended standing up with your whole body weight on one leg. Periodically change foot.
- Long periods of inactivity on long train, plane, or car journeys. Get up regularly and walk around.
- Sitting on hard objects (e.g. your wallet in your back pocket).
- Standing with your child propped up on one hip for long periods of time. Periodically change sides.

→ *see pages 121–3 for stretching and toning exercises*

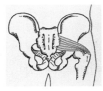

LOCATION
The anatomical location of the Piriformis muscle (above).

AREA OF PAIN
The extent of pain referral originating from the Piriformis muscle (right).

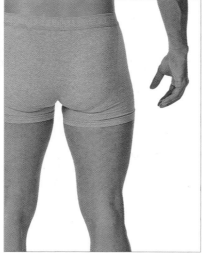

CAUSE OF PAIN: **PIRIFORMIS**

This muscle is anchored to the internal surface of the flat bone at the base of the spine (sacrum). Its other end attaches to the upper point of the thighbone. The major function of this muscle is to turn your leg outward (external rotation). It also helps lift your thigh out to the side when it is raised in front of you.

Tightness and restriction result from direct injury and chronic overload (being used too hard, for too long, too often, or any combination of these). Keep this muscle stretched and supple, especially after strenuous activity and sports.

WHAT TO AVOID:

- Twisting to the side while bending over to lift heavy objects.
- Sitting with one leg folded underneath you.
- Long periods of inactivity on long train, plane, or car journeys. Get up regularly and walk around.

➜ *see pages 140–1 for stretching and toning exercises*

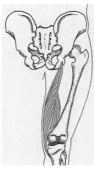

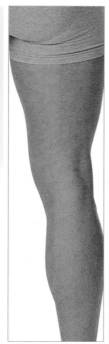

LOCATION
The anatomical location of the Semimembranosus muscle (above).

AREA OF PAIN
The extent of pain referral originating from the Semimembranosus muscle (right).

CAUSE OF PAIN: **SEMIMEMBRANOSUS**

This muscle is anchored to the bottom of the pelvis via the "sit bone" (ischial tuberosity), just behind and to the outside of the anchor points for the Bicep femoris (see page 98) and Semitendinosus (see page 121) muscles. Its other end attaches to the back of the shinbone. Contraction of this muscle bends your leg at the knee (flexion), helps rotate your thigh inward and aids in pulling it backward (extension).

Tightness and restriction can result from direct trauma (tearing or straining), prolonged shortening (from too much sitting down), or heavy, direct, and sustained compression. Keep this muscle stretched and supple, especially after strenuous activity.

WHAT TO AVOID:

- Prolonged sitting in chairs that push into the backs of your thighs (e.g. deck chairs). Choose those with rounded, well-padded front edges.
- Warm your legs up thoroughly before participating in sports that require running and jumping.

➜ *see pages 108–9 for stretching and toning exercises*

LOCATION
The anatomical location of the Semitendinosus muscle (right).

AREA OF PAIN
The extent of pain referral originating from the Semitendinosus muscle (far right).

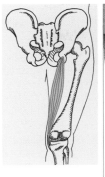
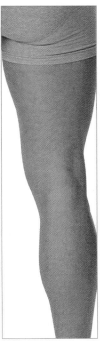

CAUSE OF PAIN: **SEMITENDINOSUS**

This muscle is anchored to the bottom of the pelvis via the "sit bone" (ischial tuberosity). Its other end attaches to the inside of the upper shinbone (tibia). The primary function of this muscle is to bend your leg at the knee (flexion). It also helps rotate your thigh inward, and pull it backward (hip extension).

Tightness and restriction can result from direct trauma (tearing or straining), prolonged shortening (from too much sitting down), or heavy, direct, and sustained compression. Keep this muscle stretched and supple, especially after strenuous activity.

WHAT TO AVOID:
- Prolonged sitting in chairs that push into the backs of your thighs (e.g. deck chairs). Choose those with rounded, well-padded front edges.
- Warm your legs up thoroughly before participating in sports that require running and jumping.

→ *see pages 108–9 for stretching and toning exercises*

LOCATION
The anatomical location of the Tensor fasciae latae muscle (right).

AREA OF PAIN
The extent of pain referral originating from the Tensor fasciae latae muscle (far right).

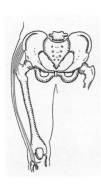
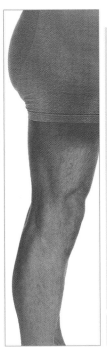

CAUSE OF PAIN: **TENSOR FASCIAE LATAE**

This muscle is anchored to the outside edge of the pelvis and to the prominent bone that juts out from the front of the hips. Its other end attaches about one-third of the way down the outer thigh. When this muscle contracts, it helps turn your leg inward (internal rotation). It also helps lift your thigh to the front, and move your leg away from your body (abduction).

Tightness and restriction can result from chronic overload and sudden or miscalculated movements (e.g. landing with a jolt after jumping or misjudging the width of a curb).

WHAT TO AVOID:
- Running on uneven surfaces, which raises one of your hips.
- Sitting with one leg folded underneath you.
- Long periods of inactivity on long train, plane, or car journeys. Get up regularly and walk around.
- Prolonged sitting with your knees higher than your hips.
- Running or jogging in sneakers with worn-down heels.
- Running or jogging without warming up and stretching this muscle beforehand.

→ *see pages 121–3 for stretching and toning exercises*

Back muscles and pain

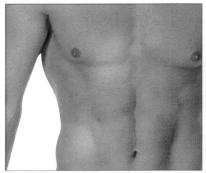

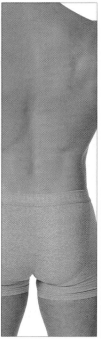

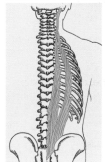

LOCATION
The anatomical location of the Erector spinae muscle (left).

AREA OF PAIN
The extent of pain referral originating from the Erector spinae muscle (above and right).

CAUSE OF PAIN: **ERECTOR SPINAE**

This group consists primarily of the Longissimus thoracis, Iliocostalis, and Spinalis muscles, and runs from the skull down to the base of the spine (sacrum). Each end of this group has the ability to move the spine, so the usual designation of "anchor-and-attachment point" is not easy to define. The primary muscles are connected to the 7th to 19th spinal vertebrae, the rear ribs, the sacrum, and the back ridge of the pelvis. When one side of this muscle contracts, it helps you bend to the side. When both sides contract, they help you lean backward and arch your back.

Tightness and restriction can result from direct trauma (tearing or straining of the muscle) and chronic overload (being worked too hard, for too long, too often, or any combination of these).

WHAT TO AVOID:
- Lifting objects without bending your knees.
- Sitting in the same position for long periods of time. Take breaks, get up, and move around.
- Sudden or awkward bending or twisting movements.
- Sleeping on very soft mattresses.

→ *see pages 110–115 for stretching and toning exercises*

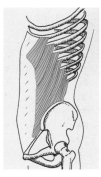

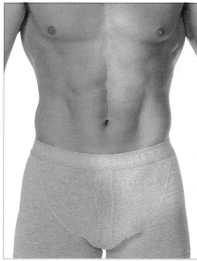

LOCATION
The anatomical location of the External oblique muscle (above).

AREA OF PAIN
The extent of pain referral originating from the External oblique muscle (right).

CAUSE OF PAIN: **EXTERNAL OBLIQUE**

This muscle covers the front side of the abdominal area and is anchored to the outer parts of the eight lowest ribs. Its other end attaches along the top front edge of the pelvis and joins to the connective tissue of the abdominal wall (abdominal aponeurosis). When this muscle contracts on one side, it helps you bend to that side and also rotates your spine. When both sides contract, this helps you bend your torso forward (e.g. when doing sit-ups). This muscle also helps support your internal organs.

Tightness and restriction can result from direct strain, chronic or acute overload (being worked too hard, for too long, too often, or any combination of these). Abdominal surgery can also cause dysfunction to these muscles (e.g. trigger points may form in, and around, post-surgical appendicitis scar tissue).

WHAT TO AVOID:
- Slouching when standing up or sitting down.
- Twisting your body when carrying heavy or awkward loads.

→ *see pages 116–118 for stretching and toning exercises*

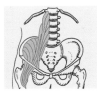

LOCATION
The anatomical location of the Iliopsoas muscle (above).

AREA OF PAIN
The extent of pain referral originating from the Iliopsoas muscle (right).

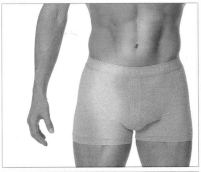

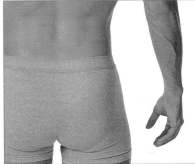

CAUSE OF PAIN: **ILIOPSOAS**

This group is a combination of three muscles. The Psoas major is anchored to the 19th to 24th spinal vertebrae and the discs in between. Its other end attaches to the thighbone. The Psoas minor is anchored to the 19th and 20th or 21st spinal vertebrae. Its other end attaches to the pubic bone. The Iliacus muscle is anchored to the inside and the top edge of the pelvis. Its other end attaches to the tendon of the Psoas major and thighbone. Contracting these muscles helps lift your thigh in front of you and assists in pulling your lower spine forward.

Tightness and restriction can result from chronic overload. If these muscles go into spasm, you may feel pain in your lower back and be unable to straighten up. Keep these muscles stretched and supple, especially after strenuous activity (e.g. gardening or sit-ups).

WHAT TO AVOID:
- Sitting with your knees higher than your hips.
- Long periods of inactivity on long train, plane, or car journeys. Get up regularly and walk around.

→ *see pages 124–5 for stretching and toning exercises*

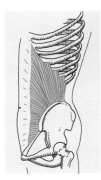

LOCATION
The anatomical location of the Internal oblique muscle (above).

AREA OF PAIN
The extent of pain referral originating from the Internal oblique muscle (right).

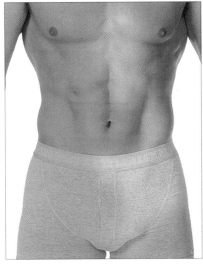

CAUSE OF PAIN: **INTERNAL OBLIQUE**

Lying directly underneath the External oblique, this muscle is anchored to the front two-thirds of the upper pelvis (anterior iliac crest), the connective tissue in the lower back (lumbar fascia), and to a ligament (inguinal ligament) that runs from the prominent bone at the front of the hips to the edge of the pubic bone. The opposite end of this fan-like muscle is attached to the last three or four ribs and the connective tissue that extends from the ribs down to the pubic bone. When this muscle contracts on one side, it helps you bend to that side and rotates your spine. When both sides contract, this bends your torso forward (e.g. for sit-ups). It also helps support the internal organs.

Shortening and restriction can result from direct strain and chronic or acute overload. Abdominal surgery can also cause dysfunction (e.g. trigger points may form in, and around post-surgical appendicitis scar tissue).

WHAT TO AVOID:
- Slouching when standing up or sitting down.
- Twisting your body when carrying heavy or awkward loads.

→ *see pages 116–118 for stretching and toning exercises*

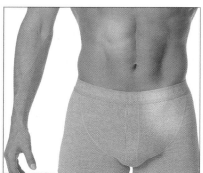

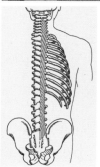

LOCATION
The anatomical location of the Multifidi muscles (left).

AREA OF PAIN
The extent of pain referral originating from the Multifidi muscles (above and right).

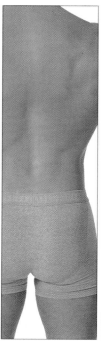

CAUSE OF PAIN: **MULTIFIDI**

These muscles run down the length of the spine and are anchored to the prominent bones on the back of the vertebrae. Their other ends are attached 2 to 4 bones down on the sides of the lower vertebrae. Contraction of these muscles helps you bend to the side (lateral flexion) and helps rotate your spine on the opposite side.

Tightness and restriction can result from direct trauma (tearing or straining the muscle) and chronic overload (being worked too hard, for too long, too often, or any combination of these).

WHAT TO AVOID:

- Lifting heavy objects without bending your knees.
- Sitting in the same position for long periods of time. Get up regularly and move around.
- Sudden, awkward bending or twisting movements.
- Sleeping on very soft mattresses.

→ *see pages 110–115 for stretching and toning exercises*

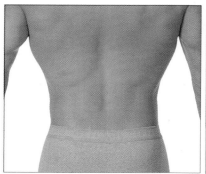

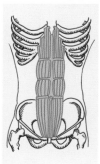

LOCATION
The anatomical location of the Rectus abdominis muscle (left).

AREA OF PAIN
The extent of pain referral originating from the Rectus abdominis muscle (above and right).

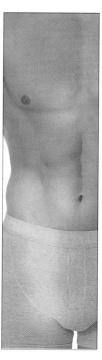

CAUSE OF PAIN: **RECTUS ABDOMINIS**

This muscle is anchored along the top edge of the pubic bone. Its other end is attached to the cartilage of the 5th, 6th, and 7th ribs at the joins with the breastbone and to the small pointed bone at the base of the breastbone. When this muscle contracts, it flexes your spine and pelvis forward (e.g. to curl up into a ball). It also helps support your internal organs.

Tightness and restriction can result from direct strain, poor posture, trauma (e.g. surgery), and chronic overload (being worked too hard, for too long, too often, or any combination of these). Keep this muscle stretched and supple, especially after strenuous activity and sports.

WHAT TO AVOID:

- Slouching when sitting down for long periods of time (e.g. while typing, writing, or reading).

→ *see page 145 for stretching and toning exercises*

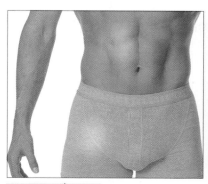

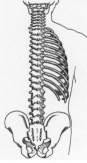

LOCATION
The anatomical location of the Rotatores (left).

AREA OF PAIN
The extent of the region of discomfort caused by pain referral originating in the Rotatores (above and right).

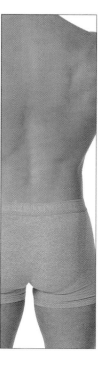

CAUSE OF PAIN: **ROTATORES**

These muscles run down the length of the spine and are anchored to the prominent bones on the backs of the vertebrae. Their other ends are attached one or two bones down on the sides of the lower vertebrae. When these muscles contract, they help rotate your spine toward the opposite side.

Tightness and restriction can result from direct trauma (tearing or straining) and chronic overload (being worked too hard, for too long, too often, or any combination of these).

WHAT TO AVOID:

- Lifting heavy objects without bending your knees.
- Sitting in the same position for long periods of time. Take regular breaks, get up, and move around.
- Sudden, awkward bending or twisting movements.
- Sleeping on very soft mattresses.

→ *see pages 110–115 for stretching and toning exercises*

Cross-referred pain

This section has been divided into the five key anatomical regions, each one capable of its own array of pain and dysfunction. At times, the line between cause and effect is not so clear. This chart will help you identify pain that may refer from one area to another.

It is possible that pain felt in a certain area is not actually caused by a tight muscle in that region but by referred pain from another, unrelated part of your body. For example, you may be experiencing pain in your shoulder but, after checking the relevant charts in the preceeding pages, are still unable to find its cause. By looking at this chart you will see that the scalene muscles are also capable of causing shoulder pain. This chart will help to shed light on some longstanding, elusive pains.

WHERE IS THE PAIN?	WHERE ELSE IT COULD ORIGINATE	OTHER CROSS-REFERRAL PATTERNS
PELVIS	Deep rotators *page 90* Gluteus medius *page 91* Gluteus minimus *page 91* Iliopsoas *page 95* Multifidi *page 96* Piriformis *page 92* Rotatores *page 97* Tensor fasciae latae *page 93*	• *Trigger points in the Rectus femoris can cause weakness in the legs, especially when walking down the stairs.* • *Trigger points can form in the Rectus femoris after hip surgery.* • *Abdominal surgery can cause trigger points to form in and around the scar tissue.*
SHOULDERS	Scalenes *page 86*	• *Trigger points in the Rhomboids can cause grating and crunching sounds when your shoulder blades move.* • *Tightness in the Serratus anterior can cause symptoms like a side-stitch during aerobic activity.* • *A tight Lower trapezius can cause the 12th thoracic vertebrae to lift, placing pressure on the nearby nerve. This can have symptoms in the stomach and small intestines.*

WHERE IS THE PAIN?	WHERE ELSE IT COULD ORIGINATE	OTHER CROSS-REFERRAL PATTERNS
HEAD AND NECK	Infraspinatus *page 77* Levator scapulae *page 78* Lower trapezius *page 78* Middle trapezius *page 79*	• *Trigger points located in the Multifidi can cause tingling, numbness, and burning sensations in your scalp.* • *Trigger points in the Splenius cervicis can cause blurred vision and eye pain.* • *Trigger points in the Sternocleidomastoid can create the classic "migraine arc" above and beside the eye socket.*
LEGS	Adductor longus *page 70* Biceps femoris *page 70* Erector spinae *page 71* Gracilis *page 72* Iliopsoas *page 95* Multifidi *page 96* Pectineus *page 73* Quadratus lumborum *page 74* Rectus femoris *page 75* Rotatores *page 97*	• *Trigger points in the Deep rotators and the Gluteus minimus can mimic sciatic pain running down the leg and into the calf.* • *Trigger points in the hamstring group can cause pain in the buttocks when you sit down.* • *Hamstring tightness is a major cause of lower-back pain.* • *Trigger points in the Gluteus maximus, Semitendinosus, and Semimembranosus muscles can cause pain in the buttocks or the coccyx when you sit down.* • *Trigger points in the Tensor fasciae latae can cause pain in the hip joint.*
BACK	Infraspinatus *page 77.* Latissimus dorsi *page 77* Levator scapulae *page 78* Lower trapezius *page 78* Middle trapezius *page 79* Quadratus lumborum *page 74* Rhomboids *page 80* Serratus anterior *page 81*	• *Whiplash accidents can cause injury to the whole of the Erector spinae.* • *Shortening of the Iliopsoas group can cause pain in the sacroiliac joint at the base of your spine.* • *Tightening of the Iliopsoas group can lead to the herniation of discs in your lower back.* • *During pregnancy, trigger points are often formed in the Iliopsoas.*

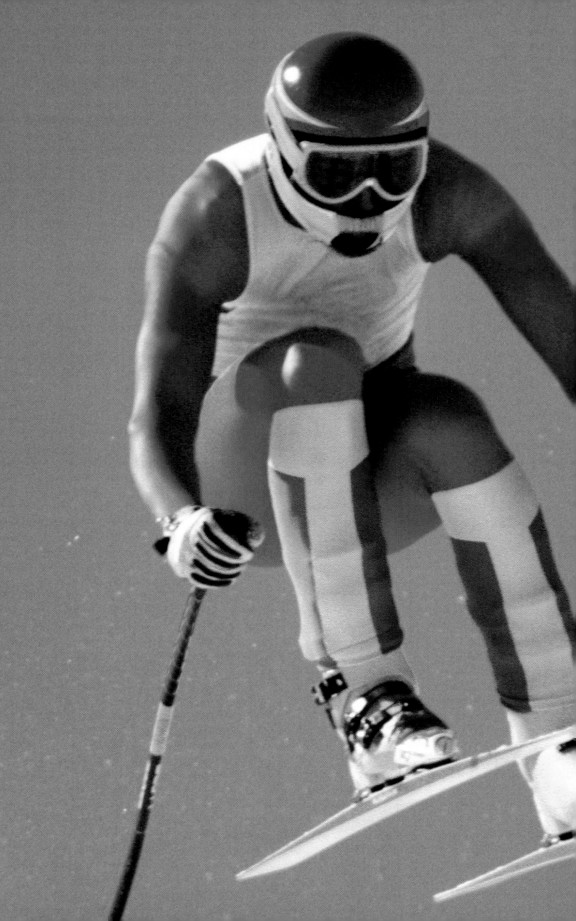

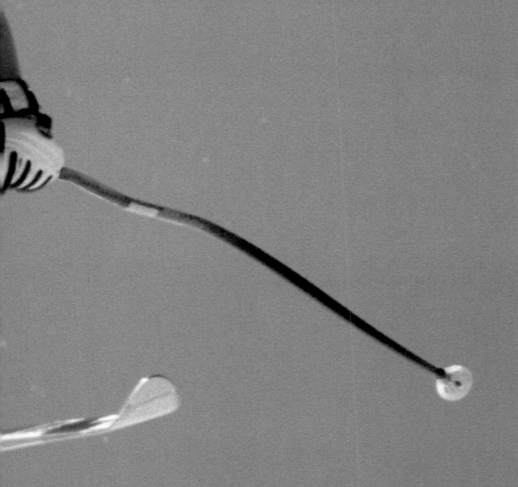

4 | **Stretching and toning exercises**

Treating imbalances

Regular stretching maintains your muscles' flexibility and is one of the best ways to safeguard against pain and dysfunction. As long as you stretch the right muscles in the right way, you'll soon feel the benefits. This section provides simple stretches to relieve tight muscles and gentle toning exercises to help even out imbalances.

The following pages include a total of 58 individual exercises that cover the needs of 48 different muscles. You don't need to do them all. Just use the body mapping section (see page 50) or the pain referral charts (see pages 70–97)—preferably both—to guide you to the exercises that suit your needs. These exercises will help you regain your postural balance and therefore your strength, stability and health.

When performing the stretching and toning exercises, stretch first and then tone. If you need to perform the stretch on both sides, stretch one side and tone the same side before you move on to the other side.

How to stretch

There are many different ways to stretch, ranging from static stretching, which involves slowly moving the muscle into a stretched position and holding that position for a set period of time—usually between 15–20 seconds—right the way through to dynamic stretching, which involves controlled and gentle swinging of your limbs.

The form of stretching that has been chosen for this book is one that requires you to contract the muscle slightly before you stretch it. This type of stretching is sometimes referred to as muscle energy technique (M.E.T.) In addition to lengthening tight, restricted muscles effectively, this type of stretching has also been shown to be a valuable tool in removing trigger points. It has also been shown to have a slight toning effect on the muscles.

Usually, when you contract a muscle it shortens in length. This shortening, in turn, moves the bone to which the muscle is attached. It is, however, possible to contract a muscle without any movement occurring. For example, imagine trying to pick up a chair that is bolted to the floor. Although the muscles in your arm would contract, the chair would not budge. This is an example of an isometric contraction (muscular force with no movement).

The interesting thing about isometric contractions is that after each contraction, the muscle automatically goes through a short period of relaxation. It is this period of relaxation that M.E.T. stretching uses to its advantage. As the muscle is more relaxed than before the contraction, it is both easier and safer to stretch.

All the stretching and toning exercises are shown on the right-hand side of the body. To perform them on the other side, simply reverse the directions. You only need to exercise the side of your body that is affected; your structural body-mapping chart should indicate whether one or both sides are affected. If both sides are affected stretch one side first, then tone, then repeat the process for the other side.

For a step-by-step guide to M.E.T. stretching, see pages 104–5.

How to tone

In Part One we touched briefly on the subject of muscle tone and its importance in maintaining a strong and stable posture, and we saw that if one muscle has become tight and restricted, it's likely that its counterpart has become weak and lost its natural tone. Each of the individual stretches in this section is followed by a toning exercise, which works the opposing muscle or muscles to the ones you have been stretching. This two-pronged approach—improving both flexibility and tone—should restore a healthy balance to your posture and will mean that your joints are protected, your physical performance will be increased, and any pain will be reduced.

The *BodySmart* toning exercises are not quite the same as the type you may be familiar with from the gym or aerobics classes. Gym-based exercises often require you to use increasing weights or resistance in order to improve your strength and fitness and to build bulk. The *BodySmart* toning exercises are gentle, therapeutic movements, in which the aim is to isolate individual muscles, contract them, and take them through their full range of motion.

When you are performing the toning exercises, concentrate on the individual muscles you are exercising so that you don't let other muscles inadvertently take over. Also, move slowly and with control; if you swing your limbs about, you'll start to use momentum, rather than the power of your muscles, and this will greatly decrease the effectiveness of the exercises.

Here are another few technique pointers you should keep in mind:

- Be careful not to overstrain your joints at any time. If an exercise requires you to work with straight arms or legs, they should be straight but not locked.
- Don't squeeze your muscles too hard or for too long. You should be able to feel the muscles working, but it shouldn't hurt. If it hurts at any time, stop and rest, then try again. If the pain is severe, stop exercising and visit your doctor.
- Breathe normally. If you find yourself holding your breath, not only are your muscles not getting enough oxygen, but it's a good bet that you're trying too hard and are beginning to overstrain your muscles.

How often should I exercise?

Perform the relevant stretching and toning exercises once or twice a day until any pain has eased and the distortion has been rectified—check your progress by repeating the body-mapping process (see pages 50–60). Then continue with the exercises for another week or two. After that you can use them every few days as part of a healthy body maintenance program.

As well as using the exercises in this book as part of a total body rebalancing program you can, of course, use the information and therapeutic exercises in this book in a more symptomatic way. If individual parts of your body are feeling tight or giving you some discomfort, check which muscles you should exercise in the pain referral charts of Part Three, then stretch and tone in the same way. Remember it's your body, so you choose.

STRETCHING STEP BY STEP

In the following example, the hamstring stretch has been used to get you familiar with the general stretching technique you will find in this book. Although the process may seem a little complicated at first glance, once you have performed these exercises a couple of times, you will find them not only easy to do but also extremely effective and rewarding. Keep referring back to this example when you first start performing the stretches in this section until you are familiar with the steps and can do them both competently and confidently.

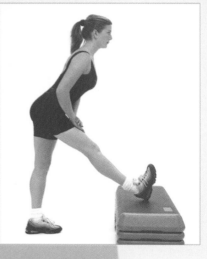

1 Stretch

Slowly move into the position of stretch. This means the point at which you are aware of a slight sensation of stretching or pulling—note the emphasis on the word "slight." Perform all of your stretches in a controlled and relaxed manner. Don't become overzealous in your pursuit of flexibility. By overstretching or placing too much pressure on the muscles, you could make them tighter and may even damage the muscles in the process. If you place too much pressure on your joints and muscles, special sensors within them react by sending a signal to your brain, which, in turn, contracts and tightens the muscles as a safety measure (see page 32, The Reflex Arc).

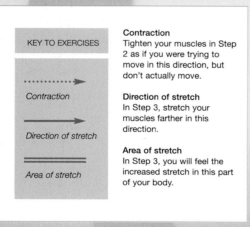

KEY TO EXERCISES	**Contraction**
	Tighten your muscles in Step 2 as if you were trying to move in this direction, but don't actually move.
Contraction	**Direction of stretch**
	In Step 3, stretch your muscles farther in this direction.
Direction of stretch	**Area of stretch**
	In Step 3, you will feel the increased stretch in this part of your body.
Area of stretch	

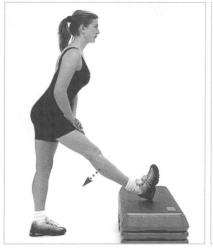 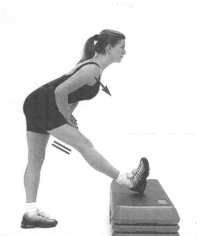

Note: This format applies to the majority of stretches in this book. However, in some cases, there are slight changes in the way the stretch should be performed. Follow the instructions carefully the first few times you perform a new exercise.

2 Ease off and contract

From this position, ease back away from the stretch until you feel the pressure on the muscles start to ease. In most cases, this should be only a very small movement of 1–2 inches (2–5 cm). At this point, you need to contract the muscles you want to stretch using no more than 20 percent of your strength. This should feel like a very gentle movement—don't squeeze the muscle as hard as you can. In this example (above), you would simply press your right heel into the exercise step. Hold this stationary contraction for 8–10 seconds.

3 Relax then stretch farther

Gently stop pushing against resistance—but don't move. It is important for the maximum effectiveness of the stretch that you simply stop contracting the muscles but maintain the same body position when relaxing.

Take a deep breath in. Exhale, slowly moving your body farther into the stretch. Once again do not overdo the stretch; just move to a position where you feel a slight stretch or restriction in easy movement. Breathing normally, hold this stretched position for 8–12 seconds.

Repeat

At the end Step 3, you have completed one cycle. Now, with the stretch you achieved in Step 3 as your new starting point, repeat Steps 2–3 another three to four times or until no improvement in the stretch is noticeable (if this happens before you have completed three or four cycles). Once your muscles have reached their limit for that particular session, it's time to stop. The amount of time you hold the positions stays the same in all the cycles (8–12 seconds). After you have completed your final stretch slowly return to a normal standing position and rest for a few seconds, before proceeding with the relevant toning exercise.

Adductor stretch
Adductor longus, Gracilis, and Pectineus

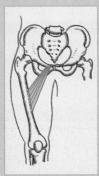
Adductor longus

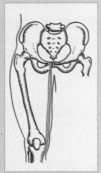
Gracilis

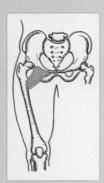
Pectineus

TIP *This exercise also stretches the Adductor brevis and Adductor longus muscles.*

KEY TO EXERCISES

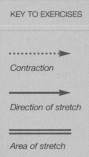

Contraction

Direction of stretch

Area of stretch

Stretching these muscles

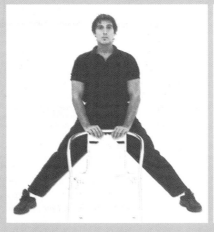

1 Place both hands on the back of a chair for support. Position your legs as far apart as is comfortable, feet facing forward.

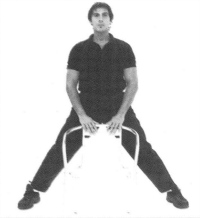

2 Bring your feet in slightly closer on either side by about 3 inches (8 cm).

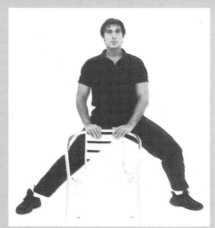

3 Keeping your right leg straight, slightly bend your left leg to the side, turning your left foot out.

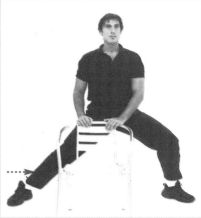

4 Gently contract your inner right thigh, as if you were attempting to bring your leg in, but don't move your leg. It should feel as if you are pushing the side of your foot into the floor. Hold this contraction for 8–10 seconds.

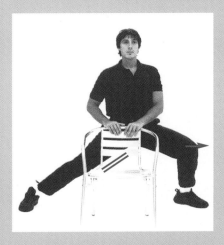

5 Relax your leg, without moving. Inhale. As you exhale, slowly move your hips to the left until you feel a slight pull on the inside of your right leg. It should feel as if you are just taking the "slack" out of the muscle. Hold for 8–12 seconds, breathing normally. Slowly allow your hips to move slightly back toward the center, just enough to take the pressure off the straightened leg. You have completed one full stretch.

Repeat steps 4–5 three or four times or until there is no increase in movement. Stand slowly and relax for a few seconds.

Toning the opposing muscles

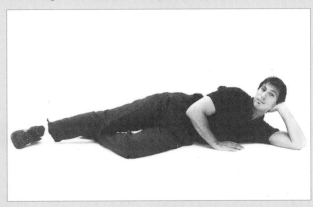

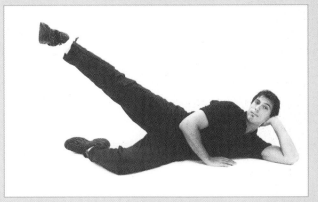

1 Lie on your left side on the floor or on a bed. Bend your left elbow and support your head and neck with your left hand. Keep your left leg comfortably folded underneath you and straighten out your right leg.

2 Keeping your right leg straight, raise it as far as you can without rotating your hips. Keep your toes pointing forward. Hold for 5–6 seconds, before gently lowering back down to the floor. Relax for a second. Repeat 8 times. Rest for 30 seconds and perform a second set of 8.

TIP Work your leg harder by keeping your foot off the floor between repetitions. Also perform a third set of 7.

Hamstring stretch
Biceps femoris, Semitendinosus, and Semimembranosus (hamstrings)

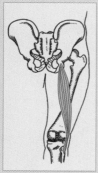

Biceps femoris

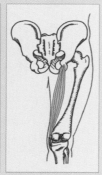

Semitendinosus

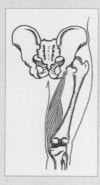

Semimembranosus

Stretching these muscles

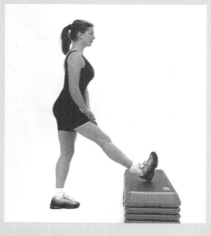

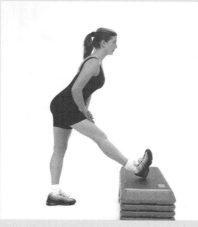

1 From standing, raise your right leg and place your flexed foot on an exercise step or low stool. Rest your hands on this thigh. Ensure your upper body is straight.

2 Check your left knee is not locked. Bend forward from your waist until you feel a slight stretch in the back of your right leg.

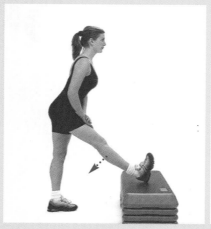

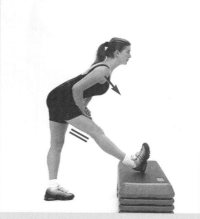

3 Ease your upper body about 2 inches (5 cm) away from the stretch to take pressure off your right leg. Then gently push your right leg down. Press your heel gently into the step or stool. Hold this contraction for 8–10 seconds.

4 Relax your right leg, without moving. Inhale. As you exhale, lower your upper body toward your right knee until you feel a gentle stretch again. Hold for 8–12 seconds. Relax, keeping still.

Repeat steps 3–4 three or four times or until there is no increase in movement. Stand and relax for a few seconds.

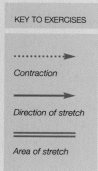

KEY TO EXERCISES

Contraction

Direction of stretch

Area of stretch

Alternative stretch

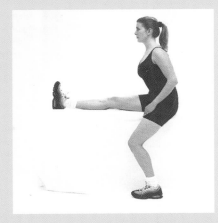 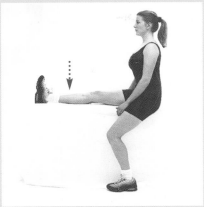 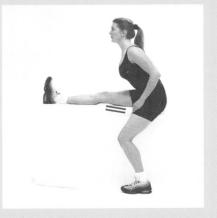

1 Sit down on the side of a low table or bed and rest your right leg straight out in front of you, foot flexed. Check your left leg is slightly bent at the knee. Keep your hands relaxed and your upper body facing straight forward.

2 Move your torso back about 2 inches (5 cm) to take pressure off your right leg. Then gently press your right heel into the bed or table. Hold this contraction for 8–10 seconds.

3 Relax, without moving. Inhale. As you exhale, lower your body forward. Don't force it. Hold for 8–12 seconds. Relax.

Repeat steps 3–4 three or four times or until there is no increase in movement. Stand slowly and relax for a few seconds.

Toning the opposing muscles

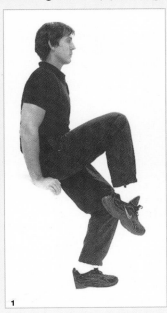 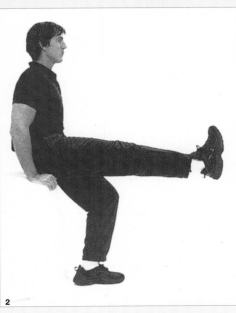

1 Sit on a tall chair or the edge of a strong table. Keeping your right knee bent, slowly lift up your right leg as high as is comfortable. Hold it there for 5–6 seconds, before slowly lowering it back down to the floor. Relax for a few seconds. Repeat 8 times.

2 From the same starting position, slowly straighten your right leg out in front. Contract the leg muscles and hold for 5–6 seconds, before gradually lowering your foot down to the floor. Relax for a second. Repeat 8 times. Rest for 30 seconds and perform a second set of 8.

TIP Make these exercises harder by keeping your foot off the floor between repetitions.

Central low-back stretch
Erector spinae, Multifidi, Rotatores

Stretching these muscles

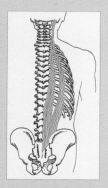

Erector spinae

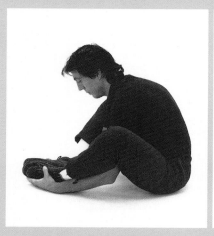

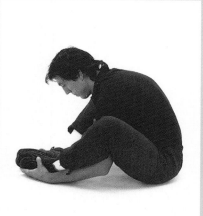

TIP *The Longissimus capitus muscles are part of this group, so are also stretched by this exercise.*

1 Sit on the floor with the soles of your feet together, knees pulled up toward your chest. Thread your hands between your thighs and under your lower legs to grasp the outsides of your feet.

2 Using your arms, pull your upper body forward and round your back until you feel a slight stretch in your back.

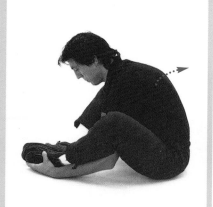

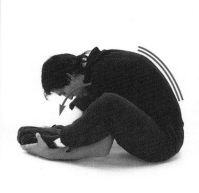

KEY TO EXERCISES

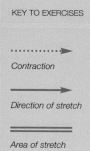

Contraction

Direction of stretch

Area of stretch

3 Ease your body slightly away from the stretch. Keep firm grasp of your feet and gently push your body backward. Use your arms to hold you steady so your back does not actually move. Hold this contraction for 8–10 seconds.

4 Relax, keeping still. Inhale. As you exhale, round your back and use your arms to pull your body forward, until you feel a gentle stretch in your back again. Hold for 8–12 seconds. Relax.

Repeat steps 3–4 three or four times or until there is no increase in movement. Sit up and relax for a few seconds.

Alternative stretch

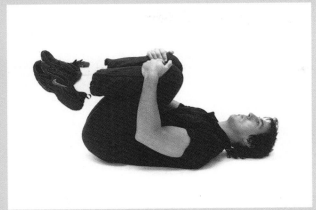 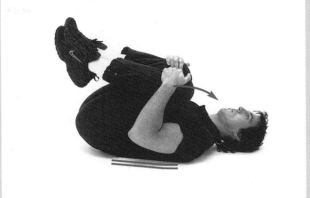

This variation is highly recommended for people with tight, restricted backs, or for people who found the stretch on the opposite page challenging.

1 Lie on your back and bring your knees toward your chest. Hold your kneecaps.

2 Inhale deeply. As you exhale, slowly bring your knees in toward your chest. Hold for 8–10 seconds. Relax and return to the starting position.

Repeat steps 3–4 three or four times or until there is no increase in movement. Lower your feet to the floor and relax for a few seconds.

Toning the opposing muscles

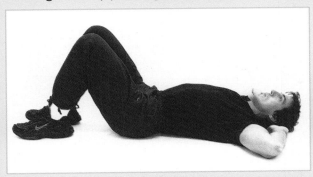 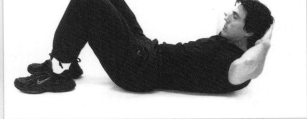

1 Lie on your back, knees bent. Position your feet flat on the floor about a foot (30 cm) away from your buttocks. Place your hands behind your head.

2 Using your stomach muscles, gently raise your shoulders and upper back off the floor. Hold for a count of two. Then slowly lower back down. Don't pull on your head at any point, your hands should just support its weight. Repeat until you have done 5–10 slow sit-ups. Rest for 30 seconds and perform a second set of 5–10 sit-ups.

> *TIP: Make this exercise harder by keeping your shoulder blades off the floor between repetitions. Also perform a third set of sit-ups.*

Central mid-back stretch
Erector spinae (lower), Multifidi, Rotatores

Stretching this muscle

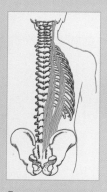

Erector spinae

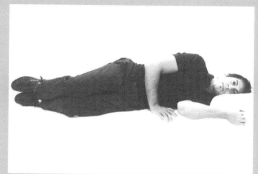

1 Lie on your left side near the edge of a bed or a large, sturdy table. Support your head with a pillow. Bend your knees.

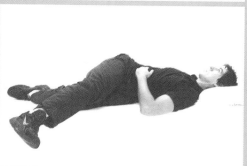

2 Keeping your legs still, stretch your right arm out to the right. Your shoulders and upper back should now be lying flat—or almost flat—on the bed or table. Straighten your right leg and move it to the left until it hangs over the edge of the bed or table and you feel a slight stretch or pulling sensation in the right of your lower back.

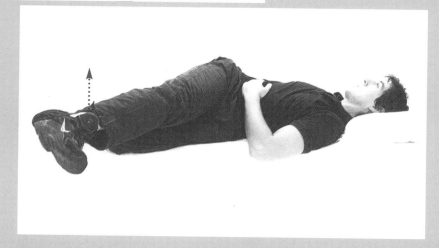

3 Keeping your right leg straight, lift it about 2 inches (5 cm) toward the ceiling. Hold this contraction for 8–10 seconds.

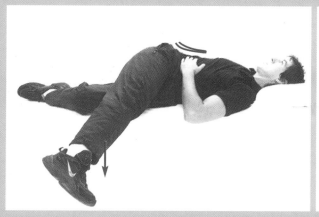 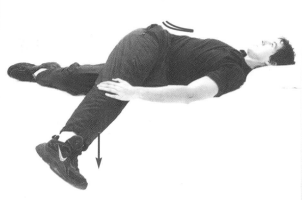

4 Inhale deeply. As you exhale, relax the muscles in your leg, and let it sink down to the left. You should notice that your leg has dropped a little farther down than it was before. Hold this stretch for 8–12 seconds. Breathe normally.

Alternatively: if you feel that you need a greater stretch, use your left hand to gently push down on your right leg during the stretching phase—do not overstretch.

Repeat steps 3–4 three or four times or until there is no increase in movement. Return to a normal lying position and relax for a few seconds.

Toning the opposing muscles

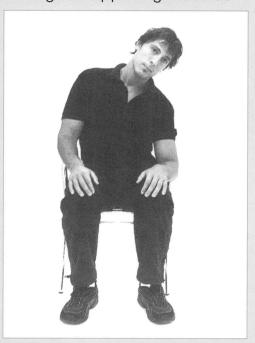

Sit on a chair. Keeping both buttocks evenly pressed down on the seat, bend your upper body to the left as far as is comfortable. Concentrate on keeping your hips level and bending from your lower back muscles. Hold this contraction for 5–6 seconds, breathing normally, then return to an upright position. Relax for a second, then repeat 8 times. Rest for 30 seconds and perform a second set of 8.

> *TIP: You may find it easier to balance if you hold the underside of the seat with your right hand.*

Central upper-back stretch
Erector spinae (upper), Multifidi, Rotatores

Stretching the muscle

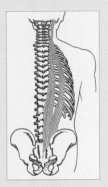

Erector spinae

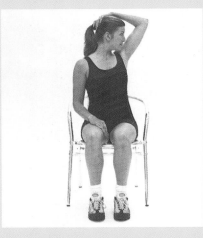

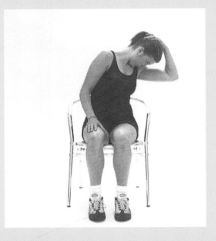

1 Sit on a chair. Turn your head to the left as far as is comfortable. Place your left hand on the top of your head, near the back. Rest your other hand in your lap.

2 Using your left hand, gently pull your head down toward your left collarbone until you feel a stretch in the base of your neck. Simultaneously bend and rotate your upper body to the left until you feel a slight stretch in the right of your back.

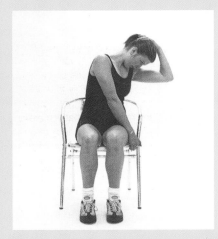

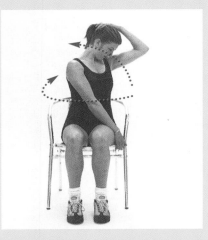

3 Bring your right arm across the front of your body and hold the front left edge of the chair.

4 Ease away from the stretch slightly. Gently contract your upper back and neck muscles as if you are trying to sit up straight, but resist the movement with your hands. Hold this contraction for 8–10 seconds.

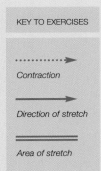

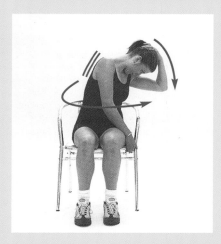

5 Relax, without moving. Inhale deeply. As you exhale, move your head farther down and increase the side-bend and rotation to the left. Do not force the stretch. It should feel as if you are just taking the "slack" out of the muscle.

Repeat steps 4 and 5 three or four times, or until there is no increase in movement. Slowly come back up to sitting and relax for a few seconds.

Toning the opposing muscles

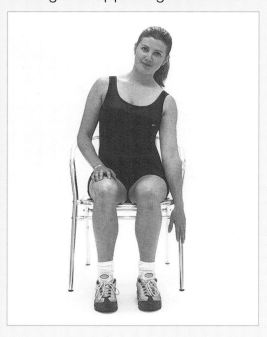

Sit in a chair. Reach your left arm toward the floor, dipping your left shoulder as far as you can. At the same time, bend your upper back slightly to the left. Imagine that your spine is straight from the base up to the middle and that you are only trying to bend the upper part to the side. Hold this contraction for 5–6 seconds, then return to an upright position. Relax for a second. Repeat 8 times. Rest for 30 seconds and perform a second set of 8.

Side stretch
External oblique and Internal oblique

Standing stretch (both muscles)

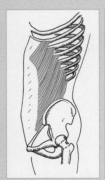 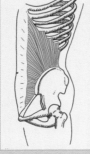

External oblique   *Internal oblique*

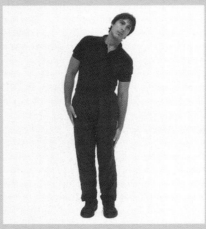

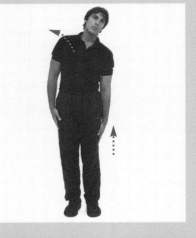

To stretch your Internal and External obliques, you need to perform two exercises for each. The first stretch is the same as for the Quadratus lumborum (see page 142). Perform this stretch first. Therefore, if you need to stretch all three muscles in the same routine, there is no need to do this stretch twice.

1 Stand with your feet about hip-width apart. Inhale deeply and, as you exhale, gently bend your upper body to the left. Move from the waist and keep your shoulders and arms relaxed.

2 Stay in this position. Inhale deeply and hold your breath. Lift your body about 2 inches (5 cm) away from the stretch. Hold this contraction for 8–10 seconds.

CAUTION: If you have a history of coronary heart disease or high blood pressure, do not hold your breath during this contraction phase.

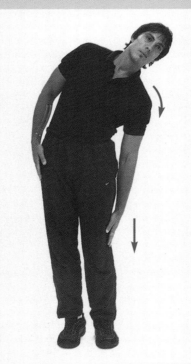

KEY TO EXERCISES

· · · · · · · · · ·▶

Contraction

──────▶

Direction of stretch

═══════

Area of stretch

3 Exhale and bend your upper body farther down to the left, sliding your hands down your leg. Do not force this movement; simply let your body relax into it. Hold for 8–12 seconds. Breathe deeply.

Repeat steps 2–3 three or four times, or there is no increase in movement. Slowly come back up to standing. Relax for a few seconds.

Alternative lying-down stretch (both muscles)

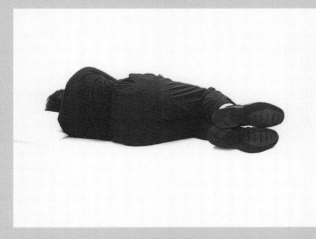

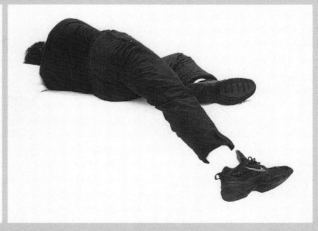

If you prefer, stretch both Oblique muscles in the following way:

1 Lie on your left side on a bed or a strong table. Position yourself diagonally across it with your legs bent for stability. Support your head with a pillow.

2 Position your buttocks as close as possible to the edge of the bed or table without losing your balance. Straighten your right leg and swing it out behind you so that it hangs off the bed or table. If necessary, grab the edge of the bed or table to help you balance.

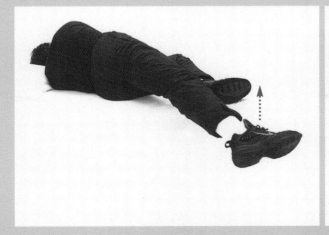
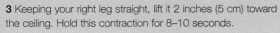

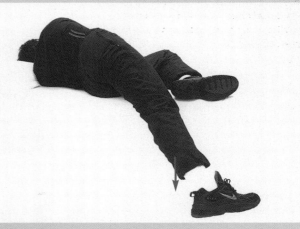

3 Keeping your right leg straight, lift it 2 inches (5 cm) toward the ceiling. Hold this contraction for 8–10 seconds.

4 Inhale deeply. As you exhale, let your leg relax completely and allow it to sink a little farther. Do not force the leg down; just let the weight of your leg and gravity pull it toward the floor. Hold for 8–12 seconds.

Repeat steps 3–4 three or four times, or until there is no increase in movement. Slowly return to lying on your side. Relax for a few seconds, before standing up.

Standing stretch (External oblique)

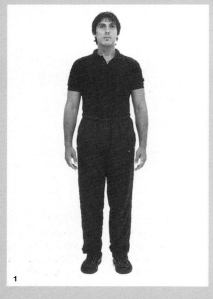
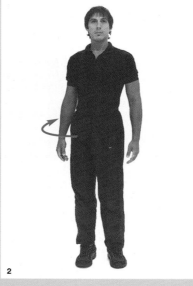

1 Stand with your feet slightly apart and your knees slightly bent. Let your arms hang loosely by your sides.

2 Inhale deeply. As you exhale, rotate your right hip backward without twisting your shoulders. Hold for 8–12 seconds. Relax, returning to the starting position. Rest for a few seconds.

Repeat the stretch three or four times, rotating your hip a little more each time.

Standing stretch (Internal oblique)

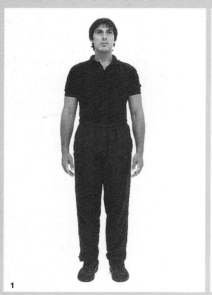
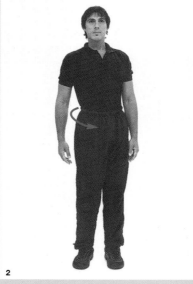

1 Stand with your feet slightly apart and your knees slightly bent. Let your arms hang loosely by your sides.

2 Inhale deeply. As you exhale, rotate your right hip forward without twisting your shoulders. Hold for 8–12 seconds. Relax, returning to the starting position. Rest for a few seconds.

Repeat the stretch three or four times, rotating your hip a little more each time.

There is no need to perform toning exercises for the opposing muscles. To rectify a horizontal pelvic twist (pelvis D), these stretches will simultaneously tone the opposing muscles. To rectify a lateral pelvic tilt (pelvis A), the toning exercise for the Quadratus lumborum on page 144 will also help to tone opposing muscles.

Buttock stretch
Gluteus maximus

Stretching this muscle

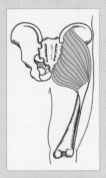

Gluteus maximus

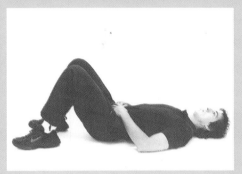

1 Lie on your back with your knees bent and your feet flat on the floor, your heels about 1 foot (30 cm) away from your buttocks.

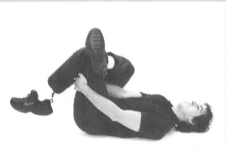

2 Rest your right ankle on your left leg, just below the knee. Keeping your head and your upper back firmly on the floor, reach forward and take hold of the back of your left thigh with both hands. Bring your left leg toward you until you feel a slight stretching or pulling sensation in and around your right buttock.

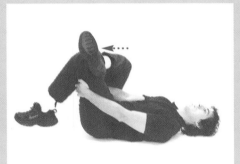

3 Move your legs back toward to the floor slightly, just enough to take pressure off your right buttock. Gently push your right leg away from you but resist the movement with your left leg, so your right leg does not actually move. Hold this contraction for 8–10 seconds.

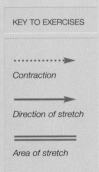

KEY TO EXERCISES

Contraction

Direction of stretch

Area of stretch

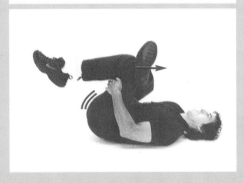

4 Relax, but don't move. Inhale deeply. Exhale, bringing your left leg toward you until you feel the stretch in your buttock again. Don't force this movement; allow the weight of your legs to do the stretch. Hold for 8–12 seconds. Breathe normally.

Repeat steps 3–4 three or four times, or until there is no increase in movement. Place your feet on the floor. Rest for a few seconds.

Toning the opposing muscles

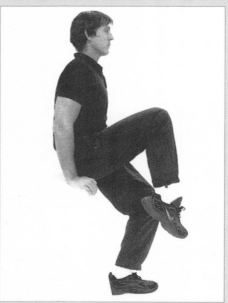

Sit on a tall chair or the edge of a strong table. Keeping your knees bent, slowly lift your right leg up as high as is comfortable and hold it there for 5–6 seconds. Slowly lower your leg back down to the floor. Relax for a second. Repeat 8 times. Rest for 30 seconds and perform a second set of 8.

TIP: Make this exercise harder by keeping your foot off the ground between repetitions. Also perform a third set of 8.

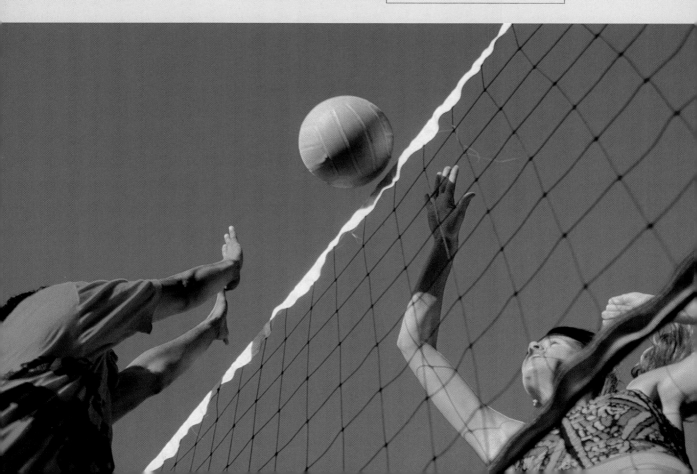

Glute/hip stretch
Gluteus medius, Gluteus minimus, and Tensor fasciae latae

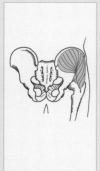

Gluteus medius

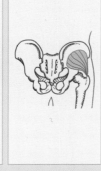

Gluteus minimus

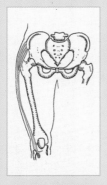

Tensor fasciae latae

KEY TO EXERCISES

········▶

Contraction

───▶

Direction of stretch

═══

Area of stretch

Stretching these muscles

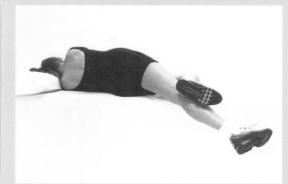

1 Lie down on a strong table or a firm bed on your left side. Support your head with a pillow. Bend your left leg. Keep your right leg straight and allow it to hang over the edge. Place your left foot on top of your right knee. Relax and allow your right leg to lower without using any force.

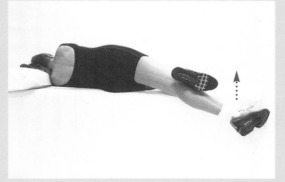

2 Keeping the same position, gently lift your right leg two inches (5 cm) toward the ceiling. Hold this contraction for 8–10 seconds.

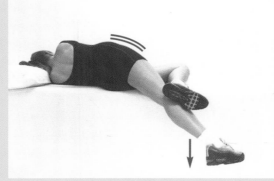

3 Inhale deeply. As you exhale, allow your right leg to lower toward the floor again without using any force. It should sink a little lower than it did before. Hold for 8–12 seconds. Breathe normally.

Repeat steps 2–3 three or four times, or until there is no increase in movement. Slowly curl up and lay on your side. Relax for a few seconds.

> *NOTE: If your right leg touches the floor during step 3, the table or bed you are using is too low. Do the variation (see page 122) of this stretch instead.*

Alternative stretch

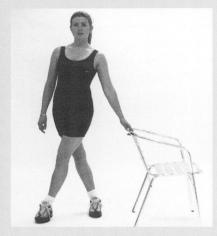 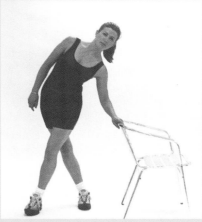 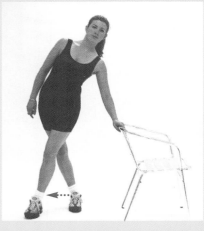

1 Hold onto the back of a chair for support. Position your right leg behind your left leg, with your right thigh touching the back of your left thigh. Place your right foot as far away from your left foot as feels comfortable, but keep both feet facing forward.

2 Keeping your feet in position, slowly bend to the left until you feel a slight stretching or pulling sensation in your right hip. As you bend sideways, do not let your body lean forward or backward.

3 Ease your upper body slightly away from the stretch, just enough to take the pressure off your right hip. Slightly bend your right leg. Gently contract your muscles as if you are drawing your right leg over to the right, but don't move your right foot. It should feel like you are pushing the side of your foot into the floor. Hold this contraction for 8–10 seconds.

4 Relax your muscles, without changing your position. Inhale deeply. As you exhale, slowly bend over to the left again. Push your right hip to the right until you feel a stretching sensation. It should feel like you are just taking the "slack" out of the muscle. Hold for 8–12 seconds. Relax, but stay in position.

Repeat steps 3–4 four or five times, or until there is no increase in movement. Slowly come back up to standing. Relax for a few seconds.

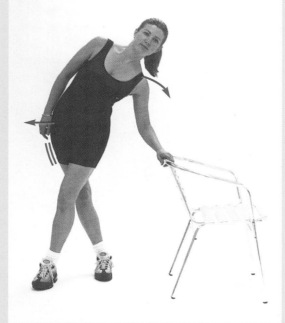

KEY TO EXERCISES

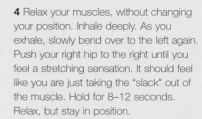

Contraction

Direction of stretch

Area of stretch

Toning the opposing muscles

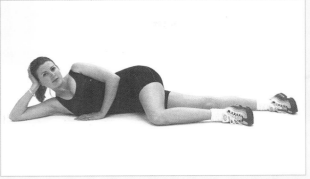 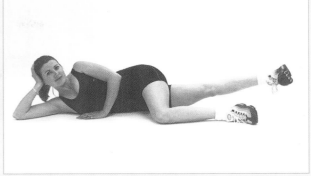

1 Lie on your right side. Bend your right elbow and support your head and neck with your right hand. Bend your left leg and rest your left knee on the floor in front of you for support. Keep your right leg straight.

2 Keeping your right leg straight, your right toes facing forward, and the inside of your right foot facing the ceiling, raise your leg as far as is comfortable. Hold for 5–6 seconds. Gently lower it back to the floor. Relax for a second. Repeat 8 times. Rest for 30 seconds and perform a second set of 8.

TIP: Make this exercise harder by keeping your foot off the floor between repetitions. Also, perform a third set of 8.

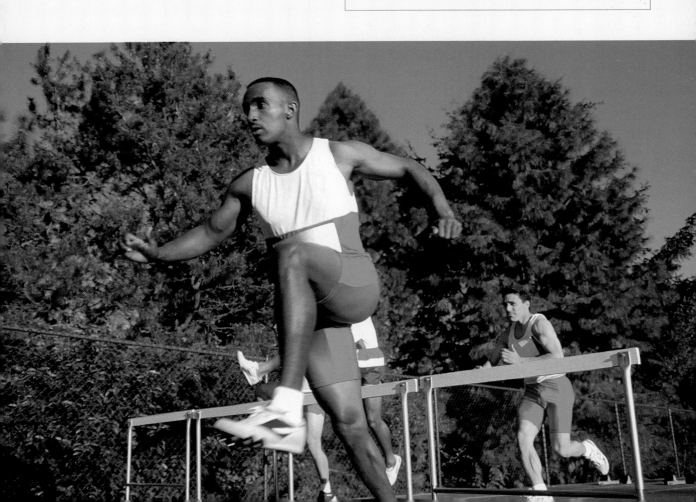

Hip flexor stretch
Iliopsoas

Stretching this muscle

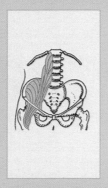

Iliopsoas

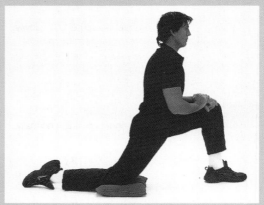

1 Place a cushion or a pillow on the floor. Kneel on it with your right knee. Keeping the top of your right foot flat on the floor, slowly move your hips and body forward until you feel a slight stretch in the front of your right thigh.

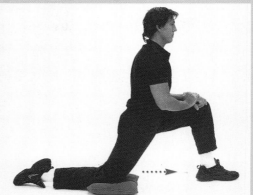

2 Ease your hips back slightly, just enough to take pressure off your right leg. In this position, gently contract the muscles of your right hip and thigh as if you are trying to pull your right knee forward along the floor. The resistance of the floor will prevent your right leg from moving. Hold this contraction for 8–10 seconds.

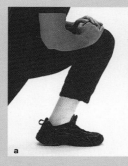

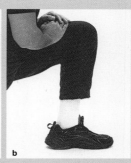

CAUTION: Your left knee should never be farther forward than the toes of your left foot (a). If this happens, reposition your left foot so your knee is behind your toes (b).

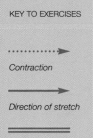

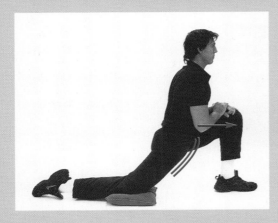

3 Relax, without moving. Inhale. As you exhale, slowly move your hips forward until you feel a slight stretch at the top of your right thigh again. It should feel as if you are just taking the "slack" out of the muscle. Hold for 8–12 seconds, breathing normally.

Repeat steps 2–3 three or four times or until there is no increase in movement. Slowly move your body back to kneeling and relax for a few seconds before standing.

Toning the opposing muscles

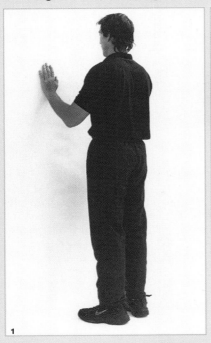

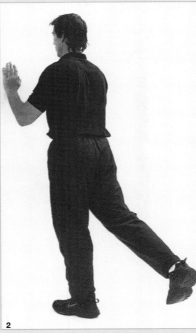

1 Stand about 1 foot (30 cm) in front of a wall. Place your hands on the wall for support and lean into it. Make sure your knees are slightly bent and not locked.

2 Slowly raise your right leg behind you as far as you can without overstraining, keeping your knee bent as you lift your foot. Hold for 5–6 seconds. Then slowly lower the leg back down. Relax for a second. Repeat 8 times. Rest for 30 seconds and perform a second set of 8.

> *TIP: Make this exercise harder by keeping your foot off the floor between repetitions. Also perform a third set of 8.*

Shoulder rotation stretch 1
Infraspinatus and Teres minor

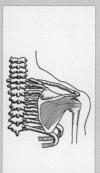

Infraspinatus

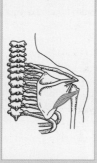

Teres minor

Stretching these muscles

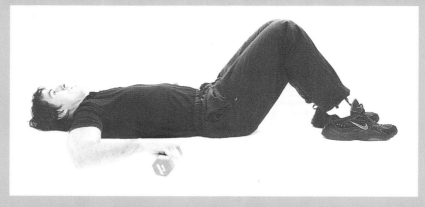

1 Lie on a bed or table with your knees bent. Hold a light weight, such as a can of beans or a dumb-bell, in your right hand. Position your right arm at 90 degrees to your right side, with your upper arm resting on the bed or table. Hang your elbow over the side and bend your elbow so that your lower arm is parallel to your body and your hand is at waist level. Let your lower arm sink toward the floor until you feel a slight stretch.

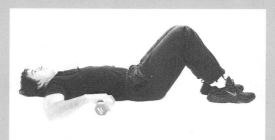

2 Pivoting only from your elbow and keeping your upper arm still, raise the weight around 2 inches (5 cm) toward the ceiling. Hold this contraction for 8–10 seconds.

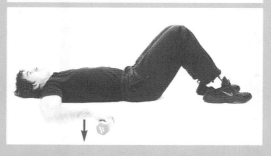

3 Gently relax and allow your right arm to drop down. Your arm should move a little lower than when you first started. Hold for 8–12 seconds. Breathe normally.

Repeat steps 2–3 three or four times, or until there is no increase in movement. Rest your arm on the bed or table and relax for a few seconds.

KEY TO EXERCISES

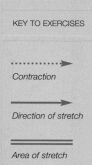

Contraction

Direction of stretch

Area of stretch

Toning the opposing muscles

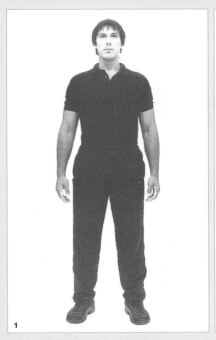

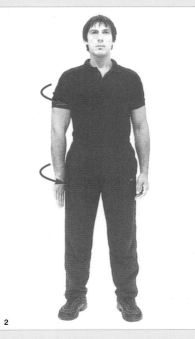

1 Stand with your feet about shoulder-width apart and your arms relaxed by your sides.

2 Rotate your right arm inward as far as you can. Hold for 5–6 seconds. Slowly allow your arm to return to its normal position. Repeat 8 times. Rest for 30 seconds and perform a second set of 8.

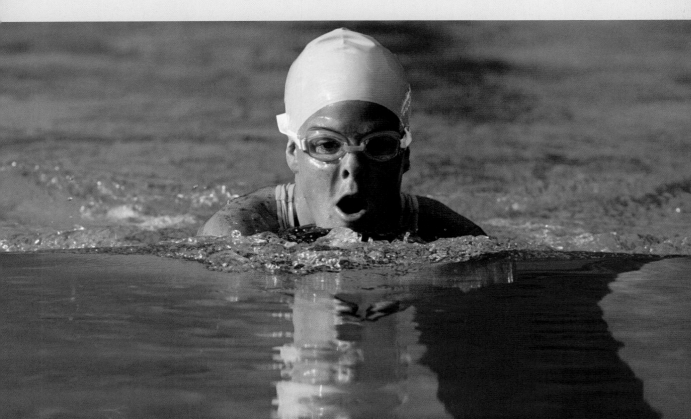

Side upper-back stretch
Latissimus dorsi and Teres major

Stretching these muscles

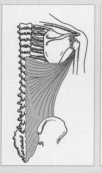

Latissimus dorsi

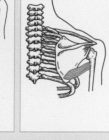

Teres major

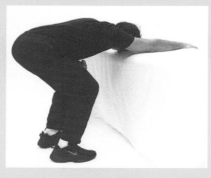

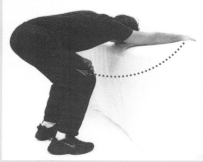

1 Find a solid table, bar, or railing at about waist level. Bend forward and take hold of the far edge with your right hand. Keeping your back straight and horizontal to the floor, slowly lean your body weight backward until you feel a slight stretching sensation along your right side.

2 Bring your upper body forward by 1–2 inches (2–5 cm), just enough to take pressure off your right side. Keeping hold with your right hand, contract your muscles as if you were trying to move your right arm in a sideways arc toward your right side. Your arm won't move, but you should feel your muscles contract. Hold this contraction for 8–10 seconds.

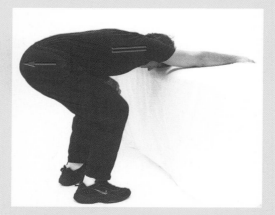

3 Relax these muscles, but stay in the same position. Inhale deeply. As you exhale, slowly lean your body weight backward again until you feel a stretch in your right side. Hold for 8–12 seconds. Breathe normally.

Repeat steps 2–3 three or four times, or until there is no further increase in movement. Release your grip and slowly come up to standing. Relax for a few seconds.

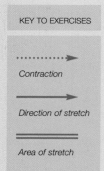

KEY TO EXERCISES

Contraction

Direction of stretch

Area of stretch

Toning the opposing muscles

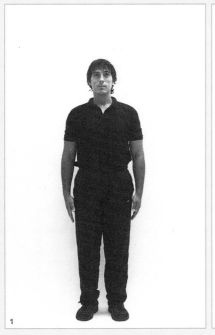

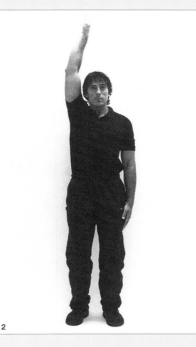

1 Stand with your feet slighty apart, your arms hanging loosely by your sides.

2 Keeping your right arm straight, raise it out to the side and bring it toward your ear, your palm facing away from you. Hold for 5–6 seconds. Reverse the movement and slowly bring your hand back down to your side. Relax for a second. Repeat 8 times. Rest for 30 seconds and perform a second set of 8.

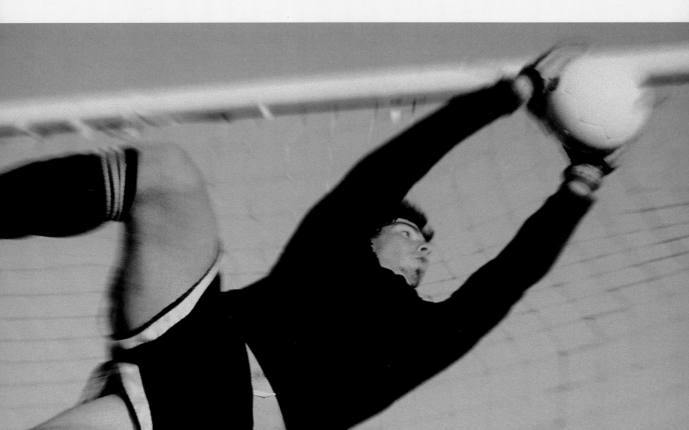

Upper shoulder/neck stretch 1
Levator scapulae

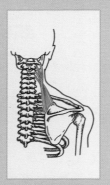

Levator scapulae

Stretching this muscle

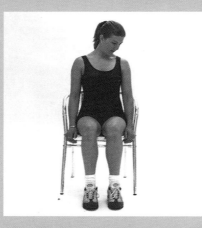

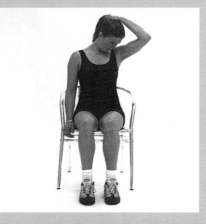

1 Sit on a chair with your hands by your sides. Avoid slouching forward or backward. Tilt your chin down toward your left nipple—until you feel a stretch in the side and back of your neck.

2 Rest your left hand lightly on top of your head. Gently use your fingertips to stabilize your head in position, but do not pull down on your head.

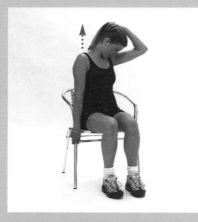

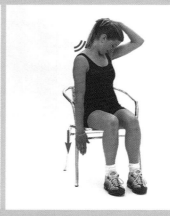

3 With your right hand, reach as far down as you can without leaning forward and grab the chair leg. Raise your head, just enough to take pressure off your neck and shoulder. Keeping hold of the chair leg, contract your muscles as if you were lifting your shoulder toward the ceiling, without letting your shoulder move. Hold this contraction for 8–10 seconds. Relax, keeping your head still.

4 Inhale. As you exhale, stretch your right arm toward the floor until you feel the stretch in your neck. Hold your head with your fingertips; avoid slouching. Hold for 8–12 seconds. Relax. Finally, lower your head a little farther toward your left nipple.

Repeat steps 3–4 three or four times, or until there is no increase in movement. Slowly straighten up your head. Relax for a few seconds.

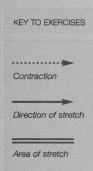

KEY TO EXERCISES

Contraction

Direction of stretch

Area of stretch

Alternative stretch

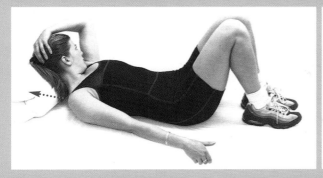 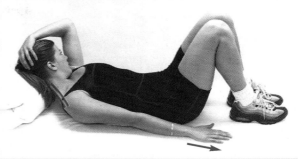

1 Lie on a firm bed or table with your head propped on pillows. Hold the side of the bed or table with your right hand. Tilt your chin toward your left nipple, until you feel a stretch in the side and back of your neck. Rest your left hand on your head and use your fingertips to keep your head still, but don't pull on it.

Ease your head back a little, enough to take pressure off your neck and shoulder. Keeping hold of the side of the bed or table, contract your muscle as if you were pulling your right shoulder up toward the pillows, without allowing your shoulder to move. Hold this contraction for 8–12 seconds. Relax, keeping still.

2 Inhale. As you exhale, reach your right arm further down the bed until you feel the stretch in the right side of your neck. Hold your head in place with your fingertips. Hold for 8–12 seconds. Relax. Lower your head a little further down toward your left nipple to take the "slack" out of the muscle.

Repeat steps 1–2 three or four times or until there is no increase in movement. Slowly return your head to a normal resting position. Relax for a few seconds.

Toning the opposing muscles

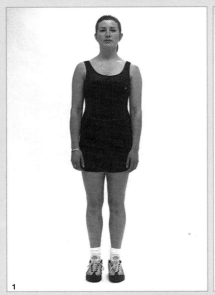 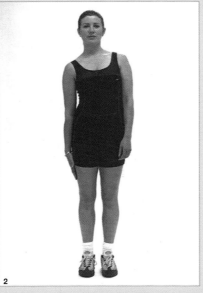

1 Stand with your feet slightly apart and your arms hanging loosely by your sides.

2 Without bending to the side, slide your right arm down your leg as if you were trying to touch the floor with your fingertips. This should only be a small movement, so don't overstrain. Hold for 5–6 seconds. Relax for a second. Repeat 8 times. Rest for 30 seconds and perform a second set of 8.

Front neck stretch
Longus capitis and Longus colli

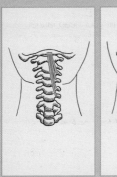

Longus capitis

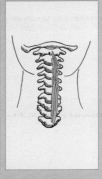

Longus colli

Stretching these muscles

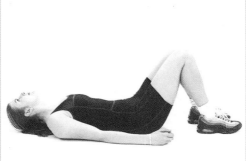

1 Lie down on the floor or on a bed. Look up and tilt your head back until you feel a slight pulling sensation in the front of your neck.

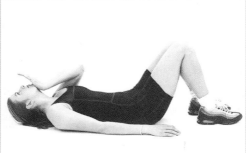

2 Place the palm of your hand against your chin.

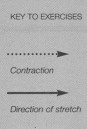

KEY TO EXERCISES

----------▶

Contraction

——————▶

Direction of stretch

═══════════

Area of stretch

3 Allow your head to come forward a little, just enough to take pressure off your neck. Gently contract your neck muscles as if you were trying to lower your chin toward your chest. Your left hand should resist the movement of your head so that it does not move. Hold this contraction for 8–10 seconds. Relax, but keep your head in the same position.

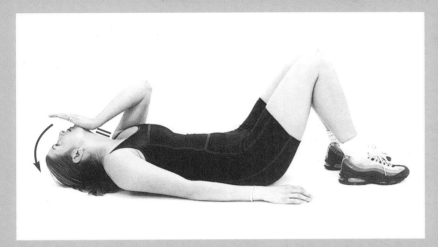

4 Inhale deeply. As you exhale, use your left hand to gently tilt your head farther back until you feel a slight stretch in the front of your neck again. It should feel as if you are just taking the "slack" out of the muscle. Hold for 8–12 seconds. Breathe normally.

Repeat steps 3–4 four or five times, or until there is no increase in movement. Bring your head back to the starting position. Relax for a few seconds.

Toning the opposing muscles

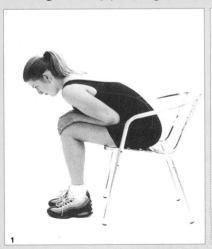

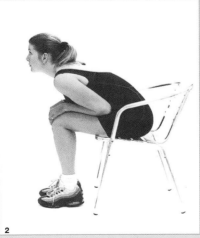

1 Sit on a chair. Keeping your back flat, bend your upper body forward until your chest almost touches your knees. Place your arms on your knees for support.

2 Lift your head and look up toward the ceiling. Hold for a count of two, then lower your head again slowly to look toward the floor. Repeat 8 times. Rest for 30 seconds and perform a second set of 8.

Side mid-back stretch
Lower trapezius

Stretching this muscle

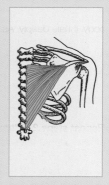

Lower trapezius

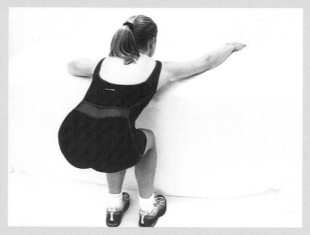

1 Find a solid table or railing that is about waist height. Keeping your back flat, bend forward. Take hold of the railing or the far edge of the table with your right hand. Make sure that your right hand is lower than your shoulder and your arm is angled away from your body at 45 degrees. Keeping a firm grip, gently lean your body away from your right hand until you feel a slight stretch in your back.

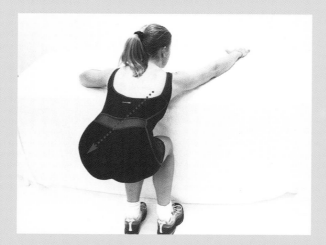

2 Ease your body forward slightly, just enough to take pressure off your muscles. Keeping a firm grasp, contract your muscles as if you were trying to pull your right shoulder blade diagonally down toward your left buttock. Your grip will prevent your arm from moving. Hold this contraction for 8–10 seconds.

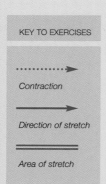

KEY TO EXERCISES

Contraction

Direction of stretch

Area of stretch

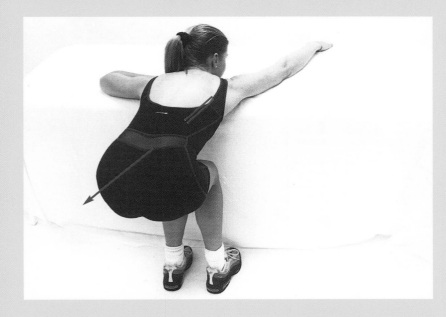

3 Gently relax, without moving your arm or body. Inhale deeply. As you exhale, slowly lean your body back diagonally, away from your hand, until you feel a stretch again. It should feel as if you are just taking the "slack" out of the muscle. Hold for 8–12 seconds. Breathe normally.

Repeat steps 2–3 three or four more times, or until there is no further increase in movement. Release your grasp, and slowly return to standing. Relax for a few seconds.

Toning the opposing muscles

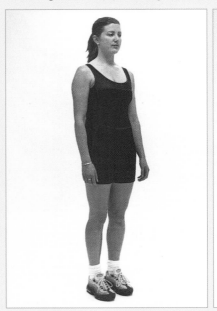
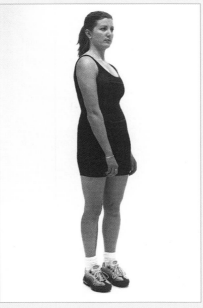

1 Stand with your feet slightly apart and your arms relaxed by your sides.

2 Push your right shoulder forward as far as you can without rotating your arm inward or twisting your upper body. Imagine you are trying to lead with the front of your shoulder. Hold this contraction for 5–6 seconds, before bringing your shoulder back to its normal position. Repeat 8 times. Rest for 30 seconds and perform a second set of 8.

Rear shoulder/mid-back stretch
Middle trapezius and Rhomboids

Stretching these muscles

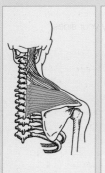

Middle trapezius

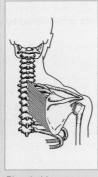

Rhomboids

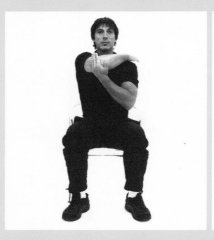

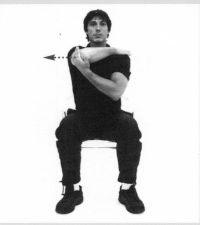

1 Sit upright on a chair and place your right hand on top of your left shoulder. Place your left hand on the back of your right elbow. Slowly pull your right elbow across your body until you feel a slight stretch in the back of your shoulder.

2 Allow your right elbow to come back slightly, just enough to take pressure off your shoulder. Gently push your right elbow against your left hand while simultaneously using your left hand to resist the push of your elbow so, although the muscle is contracting, your elbow doesn't actually move. Hold for this contraction for 8–10 seconds.

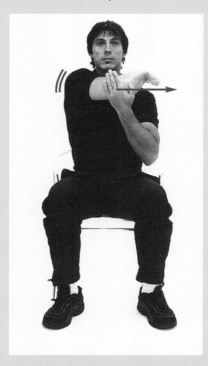

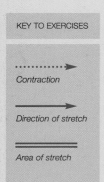

KEY TO EXERCISES

Contraction

Direction of stretch

Area of stretch

3 Gently relax, without moving your arm. Inhale deeply. As you exhale, use your left hand to draw your right elbow slowly across your body until you feel a slight stretch near the back of your shoulder. Hold for 8–12 seconds. Breathe normally.

Repeat steps 2–3 three or four more times, or until there is no increase in movement. Stand up slowly. Relax for a few seconds.

Toning the opposing muscles

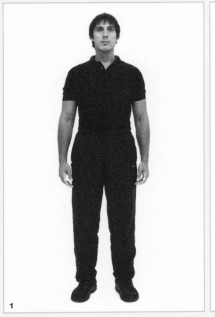

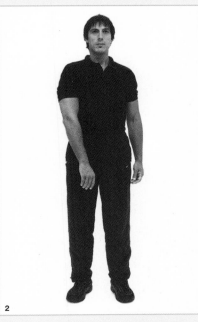

1 Stand with your feet slightly apart and your arms relaxed by your sides.

2 Push your right shoulder forward as far as possible without rotating your arm inward or twisting your upper body. Imagine you are trying to lead your body with the front of your shoulder. Hold this contraction for 5–6 seconds before bringing your shoulder back to its normal position. Repeat 8 times. Rest for 30 seconds and perform a second set of 8.

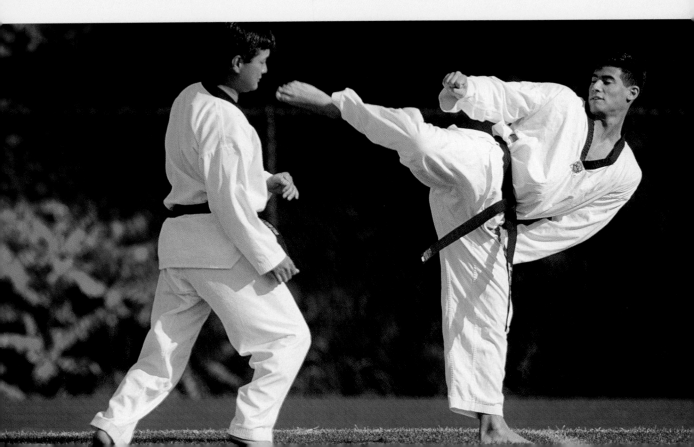

Chest stretch
Pectoralis major and Pectoralis minor

Stretching these muscles

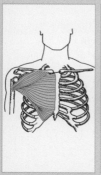

Pectoralis major

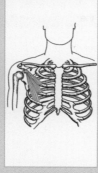

Pectoralis minor

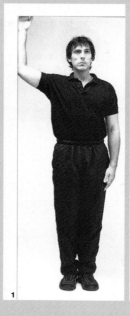

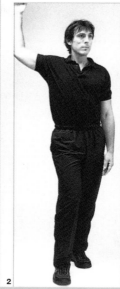

1 Stand in an open doorway with your left arm relaxed by your side. Rest your inside right forearm against the right-hand side of the doorframe. Your upper right arm should be about 45 degrees above horizontal.

2 Place your right foot slightly in front of your left. Slowly move your body forward and shift your body weight to your right leg, until you feel a slight stretch in your right shoulder and chest.

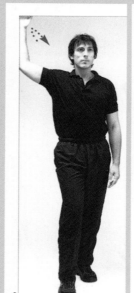

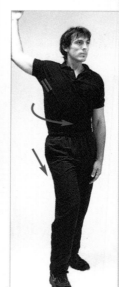

3 Ease your body back slightly, just enough to take pressure off your chest. Gently push your forearm (from elbow to fingertips) against the doorframe. Your muscles will contract but your arm should not move. Hold this contraction for 8–10 seconds.

4 Relax, without moving. Inhale deeply. As you exhale, gently lean your weight forward and turn to the left until you feel the stretch again. It should feel like you are just taking the "slack" out of the muscle. Hold for 8–12 seconds. Breathe normally.

Repeat steps 2–3 three or four times or until there is no increase in movement. Lower your arm and relax for a few seconds.

KEY TO EXERCISES

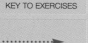

Contraction

Direction of stretch

Area of stretch

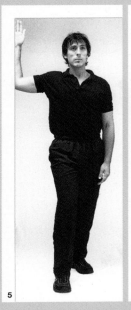

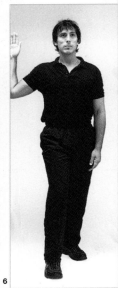

5 After your last stretch, return to the starting position, but this time adjust the position of your right arm so that your upper arm is horizontal. Repeat steps 2–4. Rest for a few seconds.

6 Return to the starting position, but this time adjust the position of your right arm so that your upper arm is about 45 degrees below horizontal. Repeat steps 2–4. Rest for a few seconds.

Toning the opposing muscles

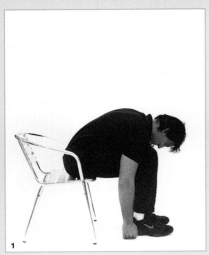

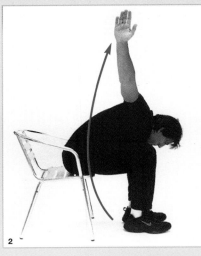

1 Sit on a chair with your feet flat on the floor. Bend your upper body so that your chest rests on your thighs. Hang your right arm toward the floor.

2 Keeping your chest on your thighs, lift your right arm out to the side and up toward the ceiling as high as you can. Hold for 5–6 seconds, before bringing your arm back down to the floor. Repeat 8 times. Rest for 30 seconds and perform a second set of 8.

> *TIP: Make this exercise harder by holding a small weight, such as a can of beans in your hand. Also perform a third set of 8.*

Rear hip stretch
Piriformis and Deep rotators

Stretching these muscles

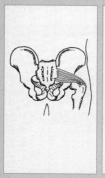
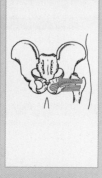

Piriformis   *Deep rotators*

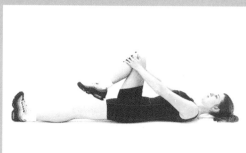

1 Lie on your back on the floor with your legs straight. Bend your right leg and bring it up, holding it without straining your neck or shoulders.

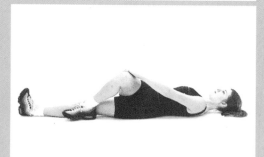

2 Keeping your lower back on the floor, place your right foot over your left knee. Using just your left hand, pull down on your right knee until you feel a stretch at the back of your right hip and buttock.

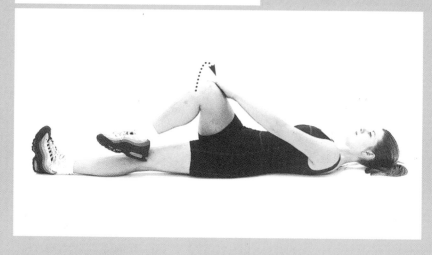

3 Ease your right knee back slightly, just enough to take pressure off your buttock. From here, contract your leg and buttock muscles as if you were trying to move your bent knee to the right, but resist the movement with your left hand. Hold this stationary contraction for 8–10 seconds.

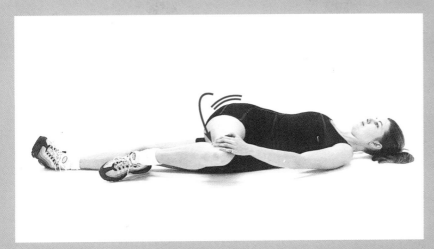

4 Relax your muscles without moving your right leg. Inhale deeply. As you exhale, use your left hand to pull your right knee farther over and to the left until you again feel a stretch in your right buttock. It should feel as if you are just taking the "slack" out of the muscle. Hold for 8–12 seconds. Breathe deeply.

Repeat steps 3-4 three or four times, or until there is no increase in movement. Slowly place your right leg back on the floor. Relax for a few seconds.

Toning the opposing muscles

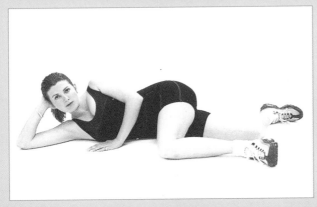

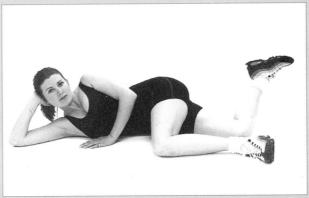

1 Lie on your right side. Bend your right elbow and support your head and neck with your right hand. Bend both your knees at about 90 degrees. Keeping the knee bent, bring your left leg forward and rest it on the floor in front of you.

2 Keeping your right thigh on the floor, slowly rotate your lower leg to raise your right foot as high as you can without straining. Hold for 5–6 seconds. Slowly lower your foot to the floor. Repeat 8 times. Rest for 30 seconds and perform a second set of 8.

TIP: To make this exercise harder, keep your foot off the floor between repetitions. Also perform a third set of 8.

Low back/side stretch
Quadratus lumborum

Stretching this muscle

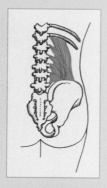

Quadratus lumborum

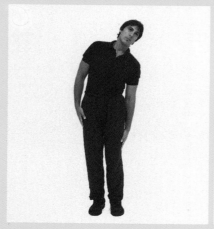

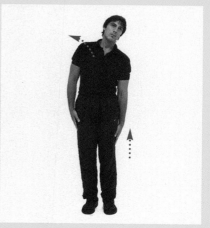

Note: This stretch is the same as for the External and Internal Obliques (see page 116). It is not necessary to repeat this stretch if you have already performed it.

1 Stand with your feet slightly apart, arms relaxed. Inhale deeply. As you exhale, gently lean your body over to the left, without straining. Keep your arms and shoulders relaxed.

2 Inhale deeply and hold your breath, as you lift your body about 2 inches (5 cm) away from the stretch. Hold this contraction for 8–10 seconds.

CAUTION: If you have a history of coronary heart disease, or high blood pressure, do not hold your breath during this contraction phase.

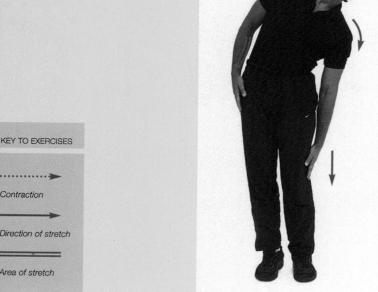

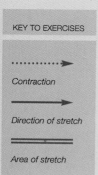
3 Exhale, allowing your body to bend over farther to the left. Do not force this movement; simply allow your body to relax into it. Hold for 8–12 seconds. Breathe normally.

Repeat steps 2–3 three or four times, or until there is no increase in movement. Slowly come back up to a normal standing position. Relax for a few seconds.

Alternative stretch

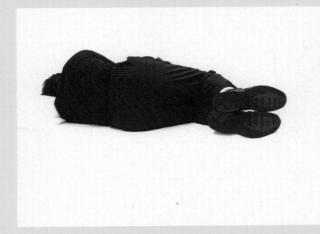

1 Lie on your left side on a bed or a strong table. Position yourself diagonally across it with your knees bent for stability.

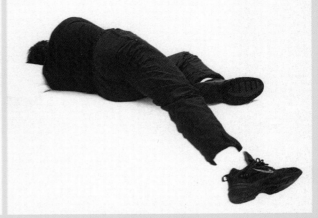

2 Position your buttocks as close as possible to the edge of the bed or table without losing your balance. If necessary, hold the edge of the bed or table for stability. Straighten your right leg and place it behind you so that it hangs off the edge of the bed or table. You should feel a slight stretch in your lower back.

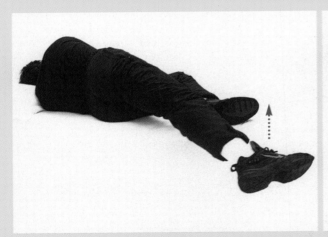

3 Keeping your right leg straight, lift it about 2 inches (5 cm) toward the ceiling. Hold this contraction for 8–10 seconds.

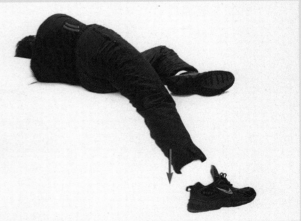

4 Inhale deeply. As you exhale, relax your leg completely and let it drop a little farther down toward the floor until you can once again feel a stretch in your lower back. Do not force the movement; just let the weight of your leg do the stretch for you. Hold for 8–12 seconds.

Repeat steps 3–4 three or four times, or until there is no increase in movement. Slowly come back up to a normal standing position. Relax for a few seconds

Toning the opposing muscles

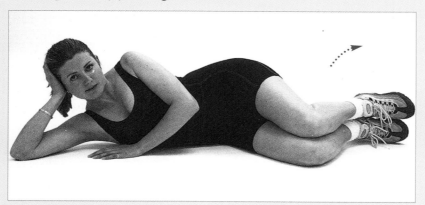

1 Lie on your right side on the floor or on a bed. Bend your right elbow and support your head and neck with your right hand. Bend your legs at the knees to help you balance.

Contract the muscles on the left-hand side of your body and attempt to lift your upper body sideways and toward the ceiling. Do not overstrain; it is okay if you cannot lift your body. You are still working your muscles by contracting them. Hold for 5–6 seconds. Relax your body back to the starting position. Repeat 8 times. Rest for 30 seconds and perform a second set of 8.

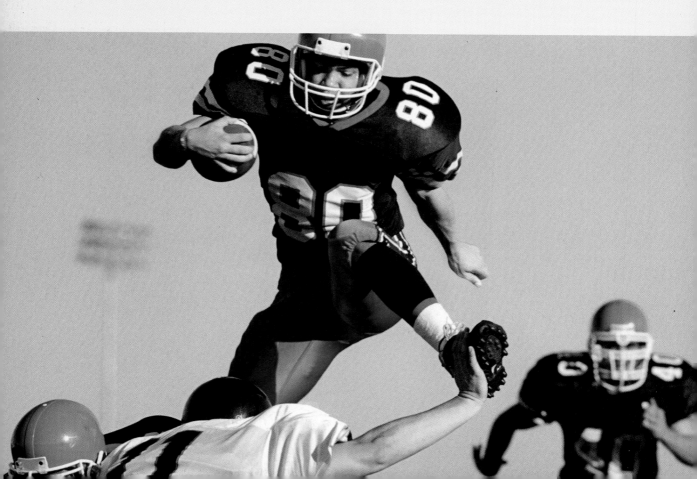

Abdominal stretch
Rectus abdominis

Horizontal stretch

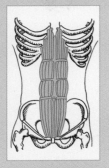

Rectus abdominis

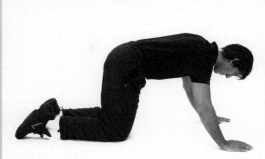

1 Position yourself on all fours with your hands about shoulder-width apart.

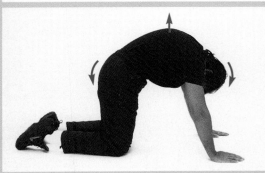

2 Tuck your chin toward your chest and curve your back toward the ceiling. Concentrate on gently contracting your stomach muscles. Hold this contraction for 8–10 seconds.

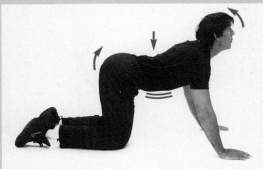

3 Inhale, arching your spine so your stomach sinks toward the floor. At the same time lift your head and pelvis toward the ceiling. Move gently; don't overstrain. Exhale, then continue to breathe normally as you hold for 8–12 seconds. If you want to increase the stretch, then without moving your hands or your shoulders pull back a little with your arms during this stretching phase.

Repeat steps 2–3 three or four times, or until there is no increase in movement. Slowly come back up to a normal standing position. Relax for a few seconds.

KEY TO EXERCISES

•••••••••••••▶

Contraction

────────▶

Direction of stretch

════════

Area of stretch

There is no need to perform toning exercises for the opposing muscles, because this stretch has the additional beneficial effect of toning them at the same time.

Rear neck stretch
Rectus capitis posterior major, Obliquus capitis inferior, Splenius capitis, and Splenius cervicis

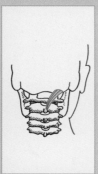

Rectus capitis posterior major

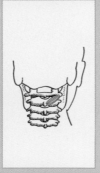

Obliquus capitis inferior

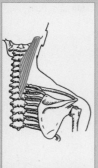

Splenius capitis

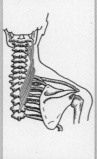

Splenius cervicis

Stretching these muscles

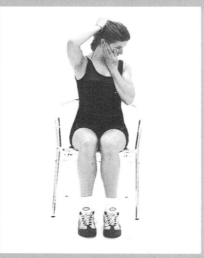

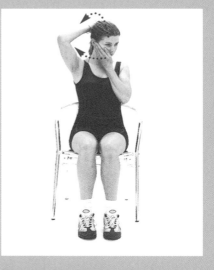

1 Sit on a chair. Rotate your head 2–3 inches (5–8 cm) to the left. Place your right hand on the back of your head and gently pull your head down until you feel a slight pulling sensation in the back of your neck. Place your left hand against your right cheek and chin.

2 Move your head back a little, just enough to take pressure off your neck. Gently contract your head and neck muscles as if you were trying to tilt your head back and to the right. Use your hands to resist these movements. Hold this contraction for 8–10 seconds. Relax, without moving the position of your head.

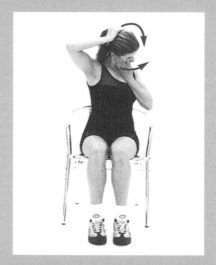

3 Inhale deeply. As you exhale, rotate your head back to the left and lower it until you feel a slight stretch in the back of your neck again. It should feel as if you are just taking the "slack" out of the muscle. Hold for 8–12 seconds. Breathe normally.

Repeat steps 2–3 three or four times, or until there is no increase in movement. Slowly bring your head back to its normal upright position. Relax for a few seconds.

There is no need to perform toning exercises for the opposing muscles, because this stretch has the additional benefit of toning them at the same time.

KEY TO EXERCISES

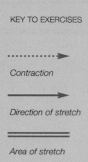

Contraction

Direction of stretch

Area of stretch

Thigh stretch
Rectus femoris

Stretching this muscle

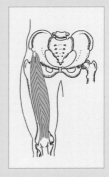

Rectus femoris

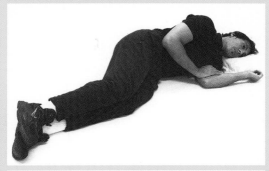

1 Lie on your left side with your knees slightly bent. Support your head on a cushion or pillow.

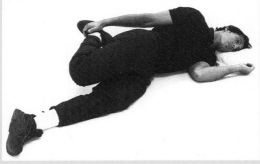

2 Take hold of your right foot and gently pull your heel toward your buttock until you feel a slight stretch in the front of your thigh.

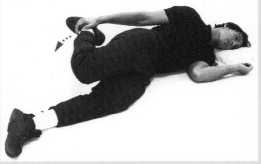

3 Ease your leg a little away from the stretch. Keeping a firm hold of your foot, gently contract your muscles as if you were attempting to straighten your leg. Resist the movement of your leg with your right hand. Hold this contraction for 8–10 seconds.

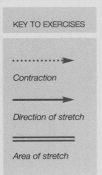

KEY TO EXERCISES

·············▶

Contraction

───────▶

Direction of stretch

══════

Area of stretch

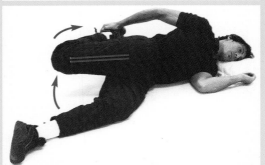

4 Relax, keeping your foot still. Inhale. As you exhale, pull your foot toward your buttock and simultaneously move your knee back until you feel a stretch in the front of your thigh. Hold for 8–12 seconds.

Repeat steps 3–4 three or four times, or until there is no increase in movement. Relax for a few seconds.

Alternative stretch

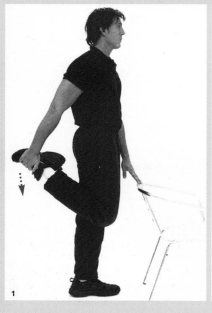 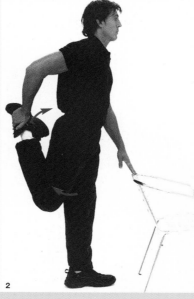

1 Stand behind a sturdy chair or close to a wall. Using the chair or wall for support, take hold of your right foot with your right hand. Pull your foot toward your buttocks until you feel a stretch in your right thigh. Move your foot back toward the floor slightly to ease the stretch. Then gently contract your muscles as if you were trying to straighten your leg, but resist the movement with your hand. Hold this contraction for 8–10 seconds.

2 Relax, keeping your foot still. Inhale. As you exhale, pull your foot closer to your buttock and move your knee back until you feel a stretch in the front of your thigh again. Hold for 8–12 seconds.

Repeat steps 1–2 three or four times, or until there is no increase in movement. Relax for a few seconds.

Toning the opposing muscles

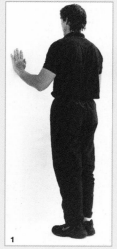 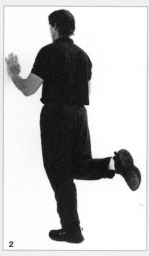 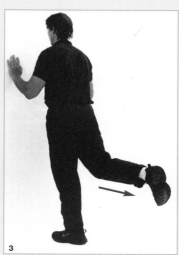

1 Stand in front of a wall with your feet together and keeping your arms slightly bent, place your hands on the wall for support.

2 Bend your right leg at the knee and raise your right heel toward your buttocks.

3 Keeping your right leg bent, slowly push it out behind you. Don't overstrain, simply push it as far back as feels comfortable. Hold for 5–6 seconds. Bring your knee forward, then place your foot back on the floor. Relax for a second. Repeat 8 times. Rest for 30 seconds and perform a second set of 8.

TIP Make this exercise harder by keeping your foot off the floor between repetitions. Also perform a third set of 8.

Side neck stretch
Scalenes

Stretching these muscles

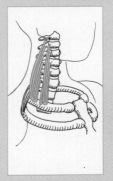

Scalenes

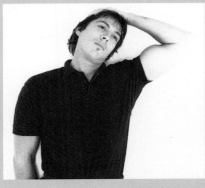

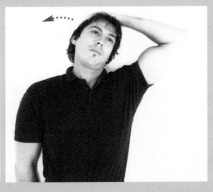

1 Lie down on the floor or a bed. Stretch your right hand down toward your feet and slide it under your leg. Tilt your head to the left as if you were trying to touch your ear to your shoulder. You should feel a slight pull in the side of your neck. Do not force the stretch. Place the fingertips of your left hand on top of your head to secure it in place.

2 Bend your head back a little to the right, just enough to take pressure off your neck. Using your left hand to resist the movement, gently attempt to bend your head back to the right. Your neck muscles will work, but your head shouldn't move. Hold this contraction for 8–10 seconds.

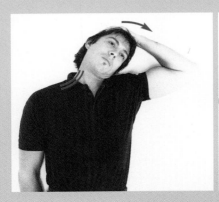

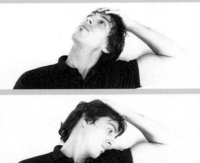

3 Relax, keeping your head still. Inhale. As you exhale, slowly pull your neck over to the left until you feel a slight stretch in your neck again. It should feel as if you are just taking the "slack" out of the muscle. Hold for 8–12 seconds.

Repeat steps 2–3 three or four times, or until there is no increase in movement.

4 Repeat the whole sequence twice more: once, starting with your chin turned to the right; and once more, starting with your chin as close to your left shoulder as is comfortably possible.

Return your head back to its normal position. Relax for a few seconds.

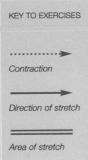

Toning the opposing muscles

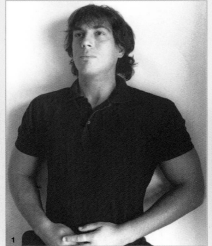 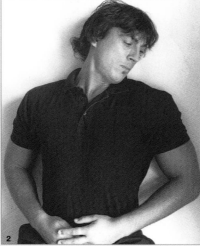

1 Lie down on the floor or on a bed. Rest your head on the floor—not on a pillow or cushion.

2 Without tensing your shoulders and arms, turn your head to the left as far as is comfortable. Then dip your chin down toward your collarbone as far as you can. Hold for a count of two.

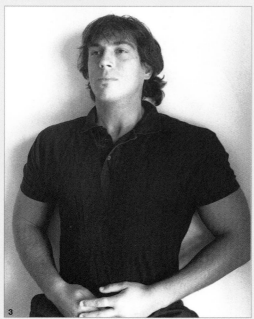

3 Reverse the movement. Lift your chin up, then rotate your head back round to the starting position. Repeat 8 times.

Central neck/upper-back stretch
Semispinalis capitis, Semispinalis cervicis, Splenius capitis, and Splenius cervicis

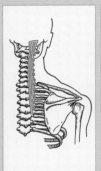
Semispinalis capitis

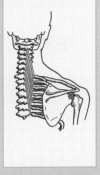
Semispinalis cervicis

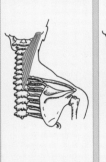
Splenius capitis

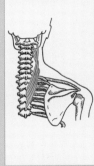
Splenius cervicis

> TIP This exercise also stretches the upper Multifidi muscles.

KEY TO EXERCISES

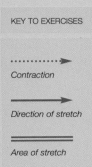

Contraction

Direction of stretch

Area of stretch

Stretching these muscles

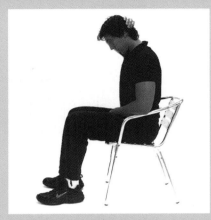

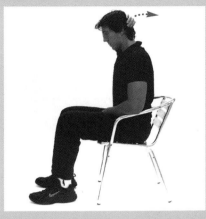

1 Sit on a chair. Place your hand on the back of your head and gently pull your head down until you feel a slight pulling sensation in the back of your neck.

2 Bring your head back slightly, just enough to take pressure off your neck. Gently contract your muscles as if you were pushing your head backward, but resist the movement with your hand. Hold the contraction for 8–10 seconds.

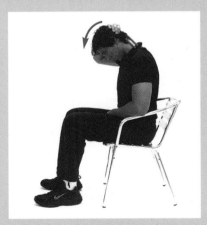

3 Relax, keeping your head still. Inhale deeply. As you exhale, gently push your head farther forward until you feel a slight stretch in the back of your neck again. It should feel as if you are just taking the "slack" out of the muscle. Hold for 8–12 seconds. Breathe normally.

Repeat steps 2–3 three or four times or until there is no increase in movement. Let your head come back to a normal position. Relax for a few seconds.

Toning the opposing muscles

Lie on your back, with your knees bent and feet flat on the floor. Inhale. As you exhale, keeping your back firmly on the floor, lift your head as if you were trying to place your chin on your chest. Hold for a count of two. Inhale, slowly lowering your head back down to the floor. Repeat 8 times. Rest for 30 seconds and perform a second set of 8.

Side torso stretch
Serratus anterior

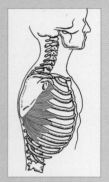

Serratus anterior

Stretching this muscle

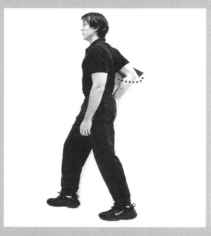

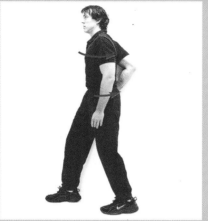

1 Stand beside a wall. Place your right hand on your hip. Press your upper arm, from shoulder to elbow, against the wall. Place your right leg in front of you for balance. Turn your upper body away from the wall until you feel a stretch or restriction. Ease away from the stretch slightly. Gently press your elbow into the wall. Hold for 8–10 seconds.

2 Relax, but keep still. Inhale. As you exhale, slowly rotate your body away from the wall until you feel a slight stretch or restriction again. Hold for 8–12 seconds.

Repeat steps 1–2 three or four times, or until there is no increase in movement. Return to standing. Relax for a few seconds.

Toning the opposing muscles

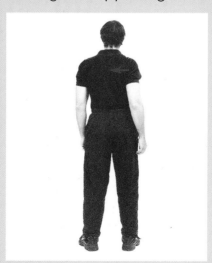

Stand with your arms relaxed by your sides. Retract your right shoulder blade in toward your spine as far as possible. Hold for 5–6 seconds, before returning to the starting position. Repeat 8 times. Rest for 30 seconds and perform a second set of 8.

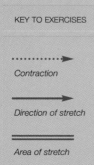

Head rotation stretch
Sternocleidomastoid and Multifidi (upper)

Stretching these muscles

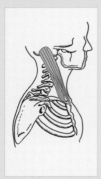 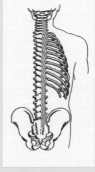

Sternocleidomastoid   Multifidi (upper)

TIP This exercise also stretches the upper Rotatores.

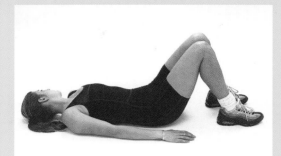

1 Lie on your back on the floor or on a bed. Turn your head to the left as far as is comfortable.

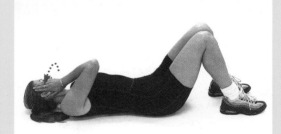

2 Turn your head back to the right slightly, just enough to take pressure off your neck. Place your right palm against the side of your face. Gently attempt to turn your head to the right, but use your hand to resist the movement. Hold this contraction for 8–10 seconds.

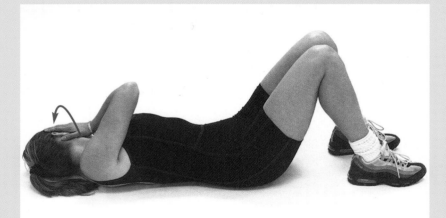

3 Relax, without moving your face or hand. Inhale deeply. As you exhale, use your hand to gently push your face to the left until you feel a slight stretch in your neck. It should feel as if you are just taking the "slack" out of the muscle. Hold for 8–12 seconds.

Repeat steps 2–3 three or four times, or until there is no increase in movement. Slowly return your head to center. Relax for a few seconds.

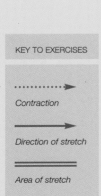

Toning the opposing muscles

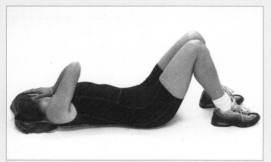

1 Lie on your back on the floor or on a bed. Turn your head to the left as far as is comfortable. Place your right palm on the right-hand side of your face.

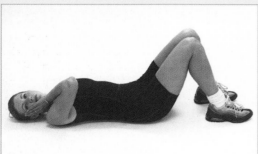

2 Rotate your head over to the right using your left hand to provide light resistance. Don't push down too hard with your hand. Turn your face as far over to the right as you can.

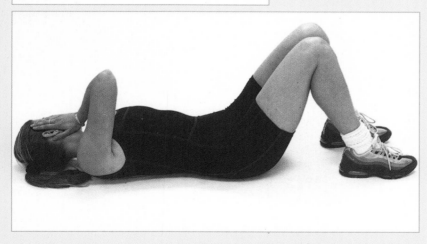

3 Bring your head back over to the left. Keep your hand pressed against your cheek. Repeat 8 times. Rest for 30 seconds and perform a second set of 8.

Shoulder rotation stretch 2
Subscapularis

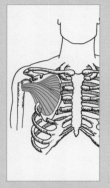

Subscapularis

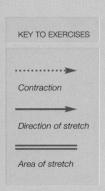

TIP *A light dumbbell or a can of beans makes an ideal weight.*

Toning the opposing muscles

1 Stand with your feet slightly apart and your arms relaxed by your sides.

2 Rotate your right arm outward as far as you can (the reverse movement of picture 2, page 127). Hold for 5–6 seconds. Return your arm to its normal position. Repeat 8 times. Rest for 30 seconds and perform a second set of 8.

KEY TO EXERCISES

........▸

Contraction

───▸

Direction of stretch

═══════

Area of stretch

Stretching this muscle

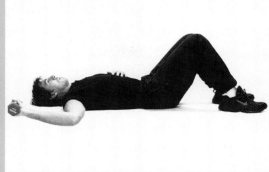

1 Lie down on a bed or table. Hold a light weight in your right hand. Position your arm over the side at 90 degrees to your body, making sure that most of your upper arm is supported. Bend your arm so your forearm is behind your head. Let your forearm drop toward the floor until you feel a slight stretch.

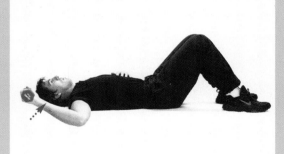

2 Pivoting only from your elbow and without moving your upper arm, raise the weight slightly toward the ceiling. Hold this contraction for 8–10 seconds.

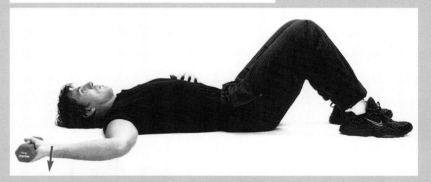

3 Gently relax, allowing your right arm to drop back down. It should have dropped a little lower down than when you first started. Hold for 8–12 seconds. Breathe normally.

Repeat steps 2–3 three or four times, or until there is no increase in movement. Slowly move your arm back down beside your body. Relax for a few seconds.

Upper shoulder/neck stretch 2
Upper trapezius

Stretching this muscle

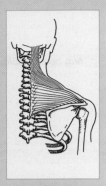

Upper trapezius

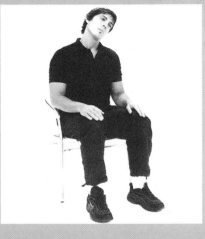

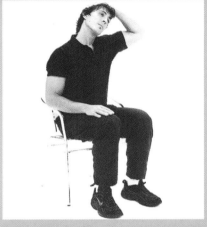

1 Sit on a chair with your back straight. Don't slouch forward or backward. Rest your hands on your thighs. Gently tilt your head over to the left, moving your left ear toward your left shoulder, until you feel a slight stretch on the right-hand side of your neck. Do not force this movement.

2 Place the fingertips of your left hand on your head to stabilize this position. Do not pull on your head.

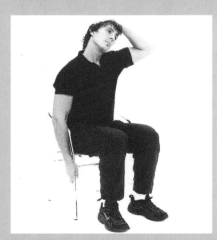

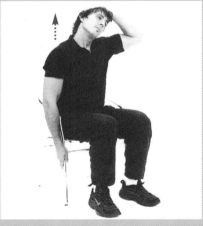

3 Reach down with your right hand and grasp the leg of the chair as far down as you can without leaning forward or moving your head. Allow your head to come back to the center slightly, just enough to take pressure off your neck and shoulder.

4 Keeping a firm grasp on the chair leg, gently contract your muscles as if you were lifting your right shoulder up to the ceiling. Your shoulder shouldn't actually move. Hold this contraction for 8–10 seconds. Relax, but keep still.

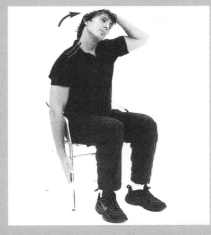

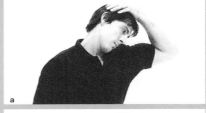

a

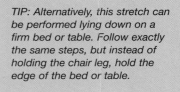

TIP: Alternatively, this stretch can be performed lying down on a firm bed or table. Follow exactly the same steps, but instead of holding the chair leg, hold the edge of the bed or table.

b

5 Inhale. As you exhale, stretch your right hand farther toward the floor until you feel a slight stretch again. Avoid slouching forward or backward. Hold for 8–12 seconds. Relax. Lower your head a little farther to the left.

Repeat steps 3–5 three or four times, or until there is no increase in movement.

6 Repeat the whole sequence twice more: once starting with your chin turned halfway toward your left shoulder (a); and once starting with your chin as close to your left shoulder as possible (b).

Slowly return your head to its normal, upright position. Relax for a few seconds.

Toning the opposing muscles

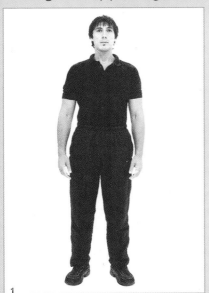

1

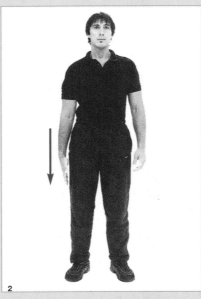

2

1 Stand with your feet slightly apart and your arms relaxed by your sides.

2 Without bending to the side, slide your right arm down your leg as if you were trying to touch the floor with your fingertips. This should only be a small movement, so don't overstrain. Hold for 5–6 seconds. Relax for a second. Repeat 8 times. Rest for 30 seconds and perform a second set of 8.

Index

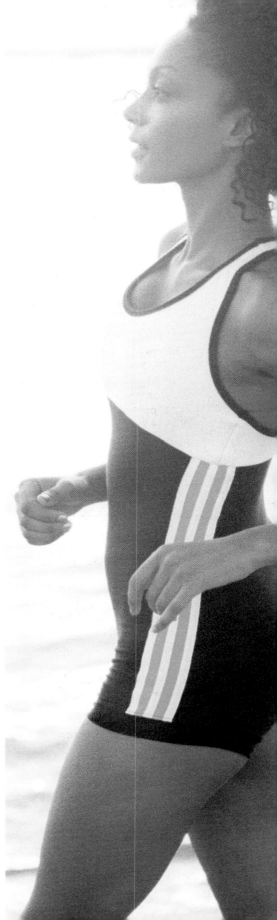

Acknowledgments

I'd like to take this opportunity to thank my many teachers, friends, and clients, who have all helped to make this work possible. Without their unique input and openness to share, this book would never have been written. Special thanks go to model Lynn Fox for her patience and professionalism, Kirsten Chapman for her sympathetic editing, everyone at Carroll & Brown for their hard work and last, but by no means least, to my partner Alison, not only for her photography but also for her constant and selfless help and support.

Just as the flames of my enthusiasm and appetite to learn were fanned by my teachers, I hope that this book will ignite your imagination, thus creating a starting point from which to discover the true nature of your physical self.

Nick Woolley

For more information on the subjects covered in this book, please visit www.body-smart.com

Carroll and Brown would like to thank:

Additional editorial work: Ian Wood
Production Director: Karol Davies
IT: Paul Stradling
Picture Researcher: Sandra Schneider

Picture credits
Page 12 CNRI/SPL
Page 14–15 Image courtesy of Reader's Digest
Page 16–17 Pete Stone/Corbis
Page 23 (right) Alfred Pasieka/SPL
Page 25 (right) Bo Veisland, MI&I /SPL
Page 29 Mehau Kulyk/SPL
Page 31 BSIP, Ducloux/SPL
Page 33 Paul Sutton/Duomo/Corbis
Page 37 Getty Images
Page 38 Getty Images
Page 56 (top right) Cristina Pedrazzini/SPL
Page 66-7 Jim Cummins/Corbis